T0244224

Sensory Healing after Developmental Trauma

of related interest

Conversation-Starters for Working with Children and Adolescents after Trauma
Simple Cognitive and Arts-Based Activities
Dawn D'Amico, LCSW, PhD
ISBN 978 1 78775 144 6
eISBN 978 1 78775 145 3

Nature-Based Allied Health Practice
Creative and Evidence-Based Strategies
Amy Wagenfeld and Shannon Marder
ISBN 978 1 80501 008 1
eISBN 978 1 80501 009 8

Raising Kids with Big, Baffling Behaviors
Brain-Body-Sensory Strategies That Really Work
Robyn Gobbel
ISBN 978 1 83997 428 1
eISBN 978 1 83997 429 8

101 Mindful Arts-Based Activities to Get Children and Adolescents Talking
Working with Severe Trauma, Abuse and Neglect Using Found and Everyday Objects
Dawn D'Amico, LCSW, PhD
ISBN 978 1 78592 731 7
eISBN 978 1 78450 422 9

Sensory Healing after Developmental Trauma

The Connected Therapist's Guide to Low-Cost Activities for Working with Children

MARTI SMITH, OTR

Foreword by Dr. Bruce Perry

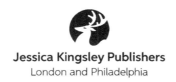

Jessica Kingsley Publishers
London and Philadelphia

First published in Great Britain in 2024 by Jessica Kingsley Publishers
An imprint of John Murray Press

3

Copyright © Marti Smith 2024

The right of Marti Smith to be identified as the Author of the Work has been asserted by them in accordance with the Copyright, Designs and Patents Act 1988.

Table 1.1 all rights reserved © 2002–2022 Bruce D. Perry

Foreword copyright © Dr. Bruce Perry 2024

Front cover image source: Michelle Nguyen.

Illustrations by Michelle Nguyen.

All rights reserved. No part of this publication may be reproduced, stored in a retrieval system, or transmitted, in any form or by any means without the prior written permission of the publisher, nor be otherwise circulated in any form of binding or cover other than that in which it is published and without a similar condition being imposed on the subsequent purchaser.

All pages marked with ✦ can be downloaded for personal use with this program, but may not be reproduced for any other purposes without the permission of the publisher.

A CIP catalogue record for this title is available from the British Library and the Library of Congress

ISBN 978 1 83997 500 4
eISBN 978 1 83997 501 1

Printed and bound by CPI Group (UK) Ltd, Croydon, CR0 4YY

Jessica Kingsley Publishers' policy is to use papers that are natural, renewable and recyclable products and made from wood grown in sustainable forests. The logging and manufacturing processes are expected to conform to the environmental regulations of the country of origin.

Jessica Kingsley Publishers
Carmelite House
50 Victoria Embankment
London EC4Y 0DZ

www.jkp.com

John Murray Press
Part of Hodder & Stoughton Ltd
An Hachette Company

Contents

Acknowledgments 6

Foreword by Dr. Bruce Perry 7

Preface 9

1. Safety, Regulation, and Resilience 13

2. Neural Networks that Connect Brain Regions 24

3. The Brainstem 31

4. The Diencephalon and Cerebellum 58

5. The Limbic Area 104

6. The Cortex 127

7. The Frontal Cortex 134

8. Assessment 147

9. Working in Different Environments 157

10. Community and Caregiver Considerations for Treatment
Planning 163

11. Practical Equipment Suggestions 166

References 200

Index 203

Acknowledgments

The very idea of this book was initiated by my guest appearance on Robyn Gobbel's podcast, "The Baffling Behavior Show [Parenting after Trauma]" (Gobbel, 2021). Robyn has been a champion for people, including me, who want to make the world a little less traumatic. You will see many references to her work in this text, because her work as a clinical psychologist specializing in supporting families impacted by trauma has influenced me profoundly, both personally and professionally. I am honored to work alongside her. You will also see a heavy influence of the work of Dr. Bruce Perry, a leading traumatologist who created a model, the NMT™ (Neurosequential Model of Therapeutics), that springboarded my journey into the world of "trauma-informed" learning in 2008. Dr. David Cross and his TBRI (Trust-Based Relational Intervention®) (TCU, n.d.) practitioner team has also been a pillar of support and guidance for me. Tracy Stackhouse, MA, OTR, especially, helped me work through much of the sensory integrative processing portions while kindly sharing her brilliance in the brain neuroscience areas. While she worked on her own projects, I'm so humbled that she found the time to assist with mine. I am so grateful to learn from each of them.

In addition, I'm so incredibly grateful for my colleagues Amy Herring Lewis, OTR, Lindsey Rachielles, OTR, Michael Remole, LCPC, and Holly Timberline, OTR, for their assistance with content and direction for this book. And lastly, thank you to all the readers of my previous book who left me comments that encouraged me to write another book.

Foreword

The human brain is comprised of more than 86 billion neurons and an equal number of glial cells, continuously interacting to create the wide range of "brain-mediated" functions. These functions range from regulatory oversight of body temperature to creating and "testing" future relational interactions with others in the mind space of imagination. From lower to higher areas of the brain, sequential, synchronous, and iterative sets of activity somehow integrate, coordinate, and create physiological, emotional, social, behavioral, and cognitive functioning. The developmental processes that lead to a fully mature, fully functioning brain involve a symphony of genetic, epigenetic, microenvironmental, and macroenvironmental factors. Considering how many moving individual cells and critical developmental steps are involved in creating a healthy brain, it is remarkable how often things go just fine. It is a testament to the redundancy, flexibility, and malleability (i.e. neuroplasticity) of the developing brain.

Neurodevelopment can be disrupted, however. A wide range of disruptive experiences and adversities can occur in utero, during infancy, and throughout childhood. These include prenatal exposure to drugs, alcohol, nicotine, stress or distress, hypoxia, or infection. Attachment experiences during infancy can be disrupted by maternal depression, domestic violence, social isolation, or even outright abuse from caregivers. Childhood can be marred by dozens of traumatic experiences, including physical, sexual, or emotional abuse, exposure to war, natural disaster, death of a parent, chronic physical illness and the multiple painful procedures that go with that, or relational rejection based on race, culture, or status. There are dozens upon dozens of potentially "sensitizing" adversities and forms of neglect. The resulting impacts on the developing brain can have catastrophic impact on the organization of key neural networks with a resulting set of functional challenges in social, emotional, cognitive, behavioral, and physical health.

For the last 40 years our interdisciplinary team has been studying the impact of these developmental adversities and looking for potential remedies. Prevention, of course, is the ideal; we all aspire to a world free of chaos, threat, racism, violence, hate, and all the collective human actions that marginalize, humiliate, degrade, and traumatize. Until that day, we must look to ways to identify (as early as possible) those impacted by developmental trauma and strive to help them. We are confident now that with developmentally appropriate educational, enrichment, and therapeutic activities, individuals impacted by neglect and trauma can begin to heal and get back on a healthy developmental trajectory. The key is relationships.

When a struggling child is lucky enough to get a clinical team that can identify their needs and strengths and put a plan in place, they will need a therapeutic web of supportive, caring, and informed adults to help provide the reparative, therapeutic moments. This is fundamentally different from the traditional medical model, which creates and reinforces the fantasy that the therapist has some unique capability to cause major change with a "magical" hour a week. This is not to demean or minimize the therapist; only to bring reality to the inefficient and often ineffective dosing schedule used by the traditional mental health therapy approach. If there is anything our 40 years of clinical and research experience teaches us, it is that the best predictor of positive outcomes is the quality and density of human connectedness.

A key feature of this therapeutic web is the developmental awareness of the caregiving environment—do the teachers, parents, or grandparents understand the child's struggles and their needs? Do they understand how to interact in simple, warm, engaged ways that will also provide the patterned, repetitive activations in the key neural networks that are under-developed or partially disorganized? To heal the child, build the tool kit and emotional capacity of the adults in the child's life. This is where Marti Smith's work can help. Practical, helpful, fun, yet therapeutic. The targeted application of sensory regulatory activities can be transformative for so many children and youth impacted by developmental trauma. This book provides a detailed overview of her interpretation of our working group's Neurosequential Model and a detailed application of specific interventions and methods to help provide the developmentally appropriate activations that can lead to healing.

Bruce D. Perry, M.D., Ph.D.
Principal, The Neurosequential Network, Houston, Texas, USA
Professor (Adjunct), Department of Psychiatry and Behavioral
Sciences, Feinberg School of Medicine, Northwestern University,
Chicago, Illinois, USA
Professor (Adjunct), School of Allied Health, Human Services and
Sport College of Science, Health and Engineering, La Trobe University
Melbourne, Victoria, Australia

Preface

This book draws from an online resource, the KALMAR app (Smith & Smith, n.d.), which I collaborated on years ago as a tool to organize brain-based and trauma-informed treatment strategies and activities aligned with Dr. Bruce Perry's Neurosequential Model of Therapeutics (NMT™). It offers questions to consider and suggests therapeutic activities to help improve brain development and function, prioritizing the lower brain regions first so that they can appropriately support higher-level brain function. In my 25 years of traveling the world and doing on-site trainings, I am often asked, "How can we continue to incorporate your ideas into our own treatment sessions after you leave us?" KALMAR was my first response to that request. This book is an expansion of that idea. It is a resource for other professionals to have a "behind-the-scenes" look at my clinical reasoning and activity selection. While it will definitely give you some "*what* to do" suggestions, I hope it also gives you an understanding of the *why* and *how* foundations of therapeutic activities.

Some of the earliest work of Dr. Bruce Perry encourages us to Regulate, before we Relate, before we Reason (Garner & Perry, 2023). The TBRI method similarly says Empower first, followed by Connection, which leads to Correction (Purvis, Cross, & Sunshine, 2007). These are all helpful ways to remind us that the brain grows, heals, and indeed functions daily on a hierarchy based on whether our needs are met and whether we care about the relationships involved in the situation. Only when we feel safe and connected relationally will any corrective or learning activity be successful.

The caregiver is responsible for the first foundations of co-regulation that later lead to self-regulation. If the caregiver isn't modeling and providing safety and connection, true behavioral change will only be temporary to ease the relational tension in that moment. Our treatment of trauma-related actions begins with the words and body language care providers use that provide true felt-safety in the situation. It begins with understanding how our past sensory experiences wired our brain based on the survivability of our earliest environments, and using that understanding to change the way we interact with individuals who experienced trauma and adversity. In order to provide trauma-compassionate and trauma-aware treatment activities, we must engage with the caregivers and help them understand brain-based function and compassion for the curious ways people who have experienced trauma and adversity may function. My dear friend and colleague, Robyn Gobbel, LMSW-Clinical, says, "Changing how we see people...changes people" (Gobbel, 2021). This phrase encourages caregivers to be empathetic to the recent learnings of neuroscience and brain imaging that prove our relational motivations are largely based on this sequential understanding. So much of our own behavior is based on predictive assumptions based on our own past experiences. When we expect the worst, that is often what we interpret. Pair this with the brain's bias towards negativity (which we indeed need to keep us safe) and we often have to work really hard to see people in a positive light.

If you have ever felt hesitation with a new client, you are not alone. I know many colleagues who wondered if they could effectively work with clients whose life experiences or trauma stirred up discomfort in themselves. I also know the majority of people, who decided to take those cases also found, like me, that they rehabbed a part of themselves in the process. In the 13th century, the Buddhist priest and philosopher Nichiren Daishonin wrote, "if one lights a fire for others, one will brighten one's own way" (Daishonin, n.d., p.1060). I urge you to light the path for the individual, the caregivers, and therefore yourself. Our lights are less likely to burn out if we continue to challenge ourselves to shine for others. Our lights shine brighter as we, as occupational therapists, can be the *related service* that helps magnify the lights of the other caregivers on our *team*.

As I have worked for the past ten years to embody this concept of changing how I see people who have experienced adversity, I have pondered how I can help with this invitation to change the way I create treatment plans. As an occupational therapist, my contribution comes in the form of activities. I desire to write content that invites the reader to understand the *how* and *why* behind the selection of activities we choose for rehabilitation of people who have experienced trauma and adversity. I believe the first step in becoming trauma responsive is to understand this very concept of how to change the way we see people. We have to first understand what happened to them and how our senses interpret those experiences uniquely based on our histories. Because *we have so much potential for our future when we can heal from our past.* For a better understanding of this concept, I recommend Dr. Perry's books (*The Boy Who Was Raised as a Dog, Born For Love, What Happened to You?*).

My hope in writing this book is to:

- Encourage you to think beyond the occupational therapy (OT) skills, on a deeper level, and see how we can inspire our clients and empower them when we add more intention and presence behind what we are doing. Be bold enough to see them as precious and worthy, despite their actions when you meet them.

- Share activities that are informed by a comprehensive occupational therapy framework while also staying grounded in the neuroscience of relationship and "felt-safety" (the deep neurological sense of feeling safe, based on our histories, combined within the context of the current moment). I believe this combination is the firm foundation of trauma-informed care.

- Give readers an inside look into how I consider OT skills within the context of the relationship with clients who have experienced adversity and traumatic events.

- Help readers formulate trauma-compassionate individualized treatment plans that are respectful and as unique as the people we work with.

CHAPTER 1

Safety, Regulation, and Resilience

We do well when we *think* we can. We engage in activities based on our current state of felt-safety and perceived ability to be successful. Occupational therapists are uniquely trained to assess the human body through many lenses, including trauma and adverse experience. We assess developmental milestones. We measure the angles of joints and tension of muscles. We bandage wounds and prevent contractures. We watch for eye movement patterns and head placement when engaged in movement activities. We assess how different types of stimulation provoke responses. When we identify areas that need improvement, we use activities that are as diverse as our clients themselves to help them and their caregivers rehabilitate those functions. To accomplish this, we must be well educated in psychology, neuroanatomy, cellular processing, physics, physical dysfunction, development, and mechanics. But, most importantly, our unique professional skill is **activity analysis**. This is the ability to look at all activities and see what foundational skill or environmental adaptations are needed to help a person be successful at any occupation or activity they desire to accomplish. Once we have identified the steps that are not coming together adequately for the client, we work sequentially to move them through the remaining steps for success in regard to that activity.

Rather than have a client continue to attempt something they do not have the skills for, I use my OT strategies of building external bracing or support to the task. This is often referred to as scaffolding the task, similar to the construction scaffolding a painter or window washer uses to reach higher locations. I adapt and support the task or activity to make it attainable. I watch to see where the child begins to disconnect or become frustrated again. Their connection to the activity usually begins to break down when their skill breaks down. A refusal to do something or even a subtle eye gaze away or excuse to move on is often my cue that this is the point where the activity needs to be therapeutically intervened. If a caregiver requests that the child clean their room and walks into the room 20 minutes later and nothing has changed, I attempt to change how the caregiver views this "disobedience." I help the caregiver have curiosity and compassion about what scaffolding the child might need to be successful rather than criticism and consequences for assumed disobedience. For most children, especially children from adversity, organization and multi-step tasks are difficult. They may not know where to begin the task. They may feel that they won't be successful or meet a standard that hasn't even been set by the caregiver. They may think "clean your room" means wash the bedding, organize all their belongings, and scrub the floor, when the intent of the directive was simply to put dirty clothes in a hamper and make the bed. They may have other things they are thinking about that are more important to their survival than if their bed looks tidy. They may have memories of past caregivers waking them up in the middle of the night and shouting at them to scrub the floor. They may have never lived in a home where there was a bed to make or enough clothes to wash.

For the majority of the people I work with, completing the task *alongside* them gives me experiential information on what parts were most difficult for them. As I work close to them, I might see something that is distracting to them. I might notice no one taught them how to put on a fitted sheet or the idea of a hamper. Maybe they never even had stuffed toys to put on a bed. This awareness helps me build a more informed relationship with them as I work to provide the skills that are lacking.

Alongside them, I can model how to make their bed while talking about how snuggly it is going to be and what great dreams I hope they will have. This approach facilitates an entirely different outcome than telling them they can't watch their favorite show until it is done and then enduring the inevitable "behavior" that will ensue because I asked them to do a task that they felt was too big and ambiguous.

The biggest therapeutic impact I can have with my clients is to walk alongside them to model and co-regulate with them as we do difficult things *together*. I like to tell my caregivers that ensuring success *with* me through our co-regulation is the key to discipline. To disciple means to lead and teach. I can't lead if I'm not *with* them. If I haven't gone back developmentally to help a client understand and practice a task *with* me, I've not *taught* them anything; I've only punished them. As we have learned with trauma research, punishment does not truly change behaviors or set an individual up for success. It sets them up for shame, robotic compliance, and avoidant lies. We need connected relational examples in our therapeutic treatments to truly have successful therapeutic outcomes. Indeed, one of the most influential courses I have ever taken that has helped me practice the art of calm presence with a foundation of neurological understanding was titled simply "Being With," taught by Robyn Gobbel (Gobbel, n.d.).

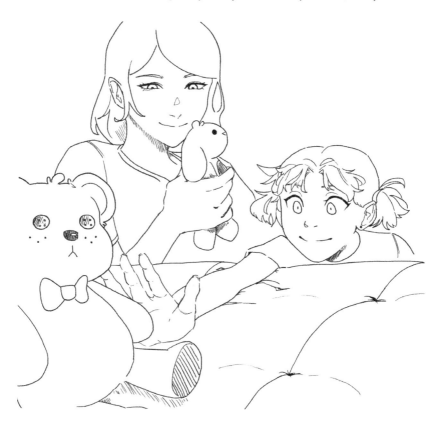

When a child can't "go make lunch," I break down the steps involved in making lunch. I become curious about whether they know what food options they have. I personally sometimes have difficulty when I open my pantry and feel like "we don't have any food" even though the shelves are full. I once saw a meme that was something to the effect of "My pantry is full, but all I see are ingredients. I can't find dinner." Often, all I see are individual ingredients without the capacity to assemble them into anything actually edible. This might be why cereal is my favorite dinner plan. I'm not always in my calm state during dinner time, when I'm thinking about who needs to be at what practice at what time and if they are ready for their big test tomorrow. Who is vegetarian today and who is on a low-carb diet? Did I answer enough emails today to close my laptop? Can that new text notification wait an hour? Seeing only ingredients without a plan or with constant distractions can be the reason my clients or I might struggle with making a simple meal. Often, this overwhelm can put us into robotic compliance, or moving through the motions without thinking, and we make not-so-healthy food choices. I might grab a bag of chips or eat an entire box of cookies. Having a pre-thought-out meal plan or a shelf with easy-to-grab healthy items that don't require thinking through nutrition labels can be a great way to support this. I aspire to some of the Pinterest boards of creating a system of drawers in the fridge where a child can choose one item from each bin to create a healthy lunch while having options that allow a sense of perceived control. But until I make that Pinterest modification in my own home, I'm likely to fall into the practiced pattern of grabbing quick and less healthy processed foods to feed my family. While I recognize that this paragraph is about highlighting the complexity of healthy eating, my hope in this section is to help you see why healthy choices are sometimes difficult, while not shaming you for doing the best you can in the moment. Some days, choosing cereal over the entire box of cookies is a win in the dietary category.

Without judgment, I can wonder if the child I'm treating had an overwhelmed caregiver who did not have the privilege of even considering nutritional content. Did they even have access to healthy options? If your veggies came from a can and you've never eaten a raw carrot, it will not occur to you to peel it or dip it in protein-rich hummus.

The texture of vegetables alone may be a completely new experience to a child who grew up with highly processed foods, which have a regulated consistency. A cracker or cookie tends to taste and feel the same with each bite. Blueberries, strawberries, and apples taste different depending on the season, growing region, and ripeness. Canned carrots require far less oral motor control than raw carrots. Processed foods are also less expensive, easier to store, and more readily available in areas of increased poverty. If a child didn't have access to fresh, healthy foods, they probably don't have a lot of practiced neural connections and motor planning on how to assemble them into a lunch box, no matter how cute the box is. Even if that caregiver asked them their favorite animal or TV show and paid extra to have a monogrammed lunch box delivered in time for the first day of school. "Packing a lunch" has many steps that need to be considered.

Once they know *what* to pack, can they open the packages independently? Do they know the steps to assemble or cook the food? Are they worried about what others will think of them when they see their food options? Are there foods inside the lunch box that will bring them happy memories or remind them of a time when things were traumatic for them? There are many things to consider when a child simply refuses to "go make lunch." Occupational therapists use activity analysis to look at the entire sequence from the request to the consumption. It is through this task that our curiosity and sequential activity analysis can lead us to intervention.

With physical challenges, we have more empathy for the lack of skill. We can *see* that someone won't be successful at a requested task. Often, we get big visual clues such as wheelchairs or orthopedic equipment. But with tasks that involve the nervous system, such as integrating various environmental sensory stimuli or cognitive skills, our own perceptions rely heavily on what we can observe. We *see* a teenager, and our own biases lead our brain to make thoughts that this teenager is capable of the task we are requesting, because we have a lot of prior experience of and exposure to teenagers being proficient at that particular problem. We need to retrain our own biases as therapists to consider what developmental milestones were not met for this teenager. What happened in their past? What experiences did they have that created learning patterns that are inefficient for a non-threatening situation? If their auditory system received a lot of adverse stimulation as a young child, their function as an adolescent will be influenced. Acutely listening and identifying the difference between a car backfiring and gunshot is a survival skill in some neighborhoods. Needing to discriminate and attune to every bang, such as a book hitting the desk, a ball bouncing in the gym, or a window closing can cause countless distractions that pull attention away from focused tasks at school.

When a child grows up in an environment where physical safety is dependent on auditory clues, their nervous system creates overly efficient connections to be on high alert for auditory input. They have difficulty filtering out the unimportant stimuli from the stimuli that fit the current context. But, as an outsider, we can't see this happening within their brain. All we see is a child who is always looking around the room, silently trying to figure out where that noise is coming from. All we see is a child who is constantly asking, "What is that noise?" or covering their ears as they try to filter out the background sounds so that they can focus on reading our facial expressions to try to figure out what we are trying to communicate to them. Or they are exhausted and need frequent breaks. Because constantly scanning the environment for cues of safety and alarm is physically exhausting.

It is important to note that mental fatigue can sometimes be even more exhausting than physical fatigue. Fatigue from physical activity tends to happen in quick bursts with time to recover between. For people who have experienced trauma, there are few breaks between the mental fatigue, and it is a more prolonged exposure. Because of this constant being "on alert," many people who experienced adversity develop an overactive stress response which is located in the "lower" brain structures such as the brainstem, cerebellum, and diencephalon. When this happens, the neural connections become very patterned and difficult to adjust without therapeutic intervention and a lot of compassion and grace for repeated practice of new neural patterning.

Adversity often wires the brain for shame and perfectionism. With trauma, an individual may have been repeatedly exposed to harsh punishments if things were not completed the way someone with power over them expected. Or maybe they only received love and attention when they performed to high standards. Either way, they have a lot of repeated neural practice with needing to be perfect, because when they weren't perfect at something, they didn't feel neurologically and relationally safe. They have negative emotions that are wired together with lack of skill that created a need for protection, the opposite of "felt-safety" (Porges, 2011). If we don't feel neurologically safe, we aren't open to trying new things and challenging ourselves. So, oftentimes, when a child doesn't have a skill for something, they move into protective mode and either run away or tear something up. This can create challenges when well-intended caregivers are trying to help them and end up feeling disrespected. Because they don't understand it is about skill, not will.

Rehabilitation happens in a sequential pattern. There must be a strong base of support before we can move forward. We must have a solid foundation and stack our building blocks in a supportive fashion to help hold up our clients. We understand that trauma impacts this sequential development. For example, if trauma happens when the eyes are developing, reading may be difficult later in life. If a toddler breaks their leg while they are learning to walk, their ability to run smoothly may be impaired without physical therapy. When an infant experiences neglect while relational attachment is developing, they may not sleep, eat, or connect with others easily.

As we assess our clients through a trauma-responsive lens, we ask what experiences they missed that could have laid the foundation for the task at hand. If a child was yelled at every time they fell, they would have a fear response to asking them to complete a complex motor sequence such as climbing a ladder and jumping off. If they lived in a crowded orphanage and were never exposed to a playground, a ladder may be completely unknown to them. They can see other children enjoying the equipment and are fearful of looking "dumb" and being teased because they have no idea how to even approach that motor skill. If a child was told "you are stupid and worthless" by a parent under the influence, they will avoid situations where they might fail. They may have self-talk that echoes those abusive comments which prevents them from even trying.

Most people do not choose to willfully disobey, challenge, or ignore the request for action. They are instead keeping their nervous system safe from perceived failure and the fear of what that has meant for them in the past. Our brains are really good at developing strategies for us to avoid continually feeling things that the brain perceives as harmful. This reframing of the *why* behind how people react to stress, requests, pressure, engagement, and challenges helps us move forward into the *what* of how to best help them fulfill their treatment goals.

In the fulfillment of those goals, we must also consider how the brain functions based on felt-safety, previous experience, and hierarchy of the brain structures responsible for task mediation.

In this book, we will explore the *why* behind some of the challenging behaviors our children show us. These are behaviors that are often labeled maladaptive and identified as needing rehabilitation, such as overreacting to small annoyances, withdrawing from loved ones, avoiding or resisting daily routines, and difficulty getting adequate nutrition. In my journey to become "trauma informed," I have been taught by trusted colleagues that children do well when they *can* (Greene, 2021). In other words, we are all doing the best we can within our capacity. So, as we look at these challenging, "maladaptive" behaviors, we remember that a thorough activity analysis is what will help us influence the behavior. We may not be able to completely change it, but we can offer hope of improvement.

State-dependent functioning is a term used by Dr. Bruce Perry (Perry & Winfrey, 2021) to explain that our functional abilities are dependent upon how stress impacts our mental state in regards to which brain system is most engaged in that moment. It is a lens through which we can better understand the child's brain-based capacity in the moment. It is how we can know what doing well "when they can" truly means for the individual *in that moment*. In Figure 1.1, Dr. Perry identifies how various parts of our brain "dial up" and "dial down" depending upon felt-safety and threat paired with our capacity to co-regulate. It highlights which primary and secondary areas of the brain are most active, and our tendency to reflect, flock, freeze, flight, or fight based on our mental states of calm, alert, alarm, fear, and terror. It also suggests how our cognition tends towards being abstract, concrete, emotional, reactive, or reflexive based on our underlying sense of felt-safety, which influences our mental state. The continuum is also used to bring awareness that people who experience adversity can have a baseline that is shifted away from felt-safety and thus moves them down the continuum even in perceived safe situations.

Table 1.1

Traditional Fight/Flight	Reflect	Flock	Freeze	Flight	Fight
Primary *secondary* Brain Areas	NEOCORTEX *Subcortex*	SUBCORTEX *Limbic*	LIMBIC *Midbrain*	MIDBRAIN *Brainstem*	BRAINSTEM *Autonomic*
Cognition	Abstract	Concrete	Emotional	Reactive	Reflective
Mental State	CALM	ALERT	ALARM	FEAR	TERROR

NEUROSEQUENTIAL
NETWORK™

All rights reserved © 2002–2022 Bruce D. Perry

When we understand how the current perceived sense of felt-safety influences the organization and immediate mental state, we can better plan our intervention strategies and work in a neurosequence that opens the more regulatory brain structures first. For example, if a person is in the mental state of alarm, we will not be able to do a magazine pictorial collage to help them determine their interests and hobbies. Their thinking and language system has been dialed down for that level of cortical processing. We also understand that someone in the mental state of terror is likely to fight and be violent, relying on reflexes to acquire a sense of felt-safety. Appealing to their emotions or even verbally communicating with them is not helpful. A better response would be to provide safety as much as possible by removing items that could be used as weapons or could result in harm to themselves or others. A person in the fear state might be able to answer direct yes/no questions, but they may not be able to have a more unfamiliar, open-ended conversation. In the following chapters, we will begin to further consider what activities are best suited for the individual as we look at their level of function through this lens of state-based functioning. In her book *Raising Kids with Big, Baffling Behaviors* (Gobbel, 2023), Robyn brilliantly expands on Dr. Perry's arousal continuum using a relational narrative format. She discusses how the nervous system can tip into owl (cortex), watchdog (arousal), or possum (dissociation). I find her book an excellent companion to this book and Dr. Perry's work.

If you are not familiar with Robyn, I highly recommend her website, podcasts, courses, and many free resources.

Resilience

After years of working with clients who have experienced trauma and adversity, I've seen my own validation of Dr. Perry's resilience versus vulnerability work (Perry & Winfrey, 2021). In his teaching, he states that when a stressor is unpredictable, uncontrollable, or severe, the individual is more likely to become vulnerable. When the stressor is predictable, controllable, and mild, the individual is more likely to become resilient. As I look at activity selection, I keep these three keys (predictable vs. unpredictable, controllable vs. uncontrollable, mild vs. severe) in mind. In order to create rehabilitative change, I often must stress the body. Some therapists might call this the "just-right" challenge. It is the ability to bring the client to the edge of their ability and then sit with them on that edge as co-regulated support to help them move towards healing.

A common goal I work towards is "sensory acceptance" such as "Patient will tolerate textures on their hands" or "Patient will tolerate moderate-level noise in the cafeteria." When I see this as a goal, I'm cued in that this client may not feel safe with certain types of sensory experiences. Maybe they violently push the sensations away or become rigid and controlling in their daily routines to avoid sensations. Using this resilience framework, I can see that they are seeking control to help decrease their vulnerability. They are using this rigid control to help the brain better predict the sensations coming in so that they can maintain an appropriate level of stress response to the stimulation. When they know what is coming, they can be more accepting of the sensation. As I develop therapeutic activity to help them habituate, better interpret, process, or integrate the sensation, I look for ways to incorporate mild intensity, predictability, and control. I don't just randomly bombard their senses. I let them know what is happening and that they can stop at any time. I allow them ways to control the intensity and duration of the sensory input. For tactile sensations, I might allow them to fill the bucket with the sensory medium them-selves or provide a "safety rag" that is wet on one end and dry on the other that they can use at their discretion. I try to increase the predictability by adding rhythm or repetition. We might sing a song while in the tactile medium or engage in the activity while swinging or listening to music. I might hide several items in the medium and we count them as they are discovered as a way to add repetition and predictive planning. As we begin to explore more treatment activities, you may also find that I lean heavily into Dr. Perry's six Rs of therapeutic activity (Garner & Perry, 2023). As you plan your treatment, ask if the activity is Rewarding, Relational, Relevant (age-appropriate and meaningful), Respectful, Rhythmic, and Repetitive. With a foundation of felt-safety and connection through relationship, these six Rs can be a great filter as you create a trauma-compassionate treatment plan.

CHAPTER 2

Neural Networks that Connect Brain Regions

As we begin to clinically reason through the neurosequential process while deciding what therapeutic activity to select, there is no way to fully limit discussion to just one brain region or mental state. Our mental states shift quickly, and our brain is *full* of complex connections. Simply articulating the word "stop" could involve every part of the brain. The brainstem might signal the alarm and raise the heart rate and breath to get the word out forcefully. The limbic system might be taking an emotional snapshot of the surroundings to understand what is happening and why we need to make the protective move of stopping something. The words are formed in the Broca's area of the left hemisphere of the motor cortex. The angular gyrus assembles information to help us understand words and concepts. Wernicke's area helps process the word "stop" to determine context and meaning. The cortex is thinking about how to proceed if the stop happens or not. The frontal cortex is sending thoughtful signals keeping the body calm so that we can simply use our words and not fists (which would be the motor cortex) to communicate our desire for something to stop. I imagine an fMRI like a fireworks show. Simply saying the word "stop" is quite the colorful light show in that brain imaging.

When Amy Lewis, OTR, told me about Lisa Feldman Barrett's analogy—that our neural connections are like air traffic controllers (Barrett, 2017)—it resonated with me. Although we are first taught a straightforward "sensory IN, motor OUT" model, the brain doesn't really function like a two-way highway where information goes up the spinal cord, hits a roundabout, and comes back down. It is organized more like major airport hubs with lots of smaller regional airfields and even a few private airstrips. Different types of sensations could be compared to different airlines. The vision airline might be hubbed in the visual cortex, but there will be smaller landing strips in the areas of the brain associated with visual memory, color, and visual motor skills. The sense of touch would be an entirely different, larger airline company with hubs in different places like the thalamus, primary motor cortex, and limbic system. This touch airline would also land in some of the smaller fields of the motor cortex that the sense of vision uses as we interpret how items we see in our hand feel. The thalamus would be one of the international major airport hubs where *many* senses come together and unload information while loading up information to take to other smaller airports.

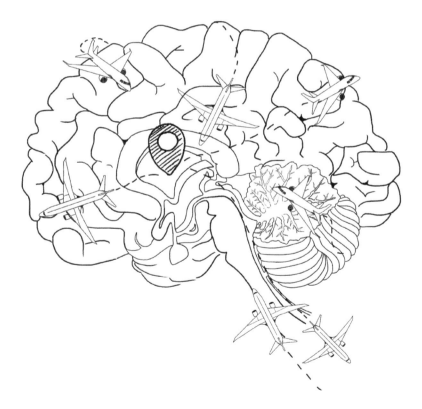

Using this analogy, we can see how the parts of our brain are intricately connected. We quickly realize that nothing happens in isolation.

Icelandair might be our math facts airline, circling around Iceland (the frontal cortex) with a few strategic international flights out to the visual spatial and working memory centers. Southwest Airlines would be our emotions hub in the insular cortex, with many connecting flights and unexpected layovers and smaller airfield stops to the areas that mediate facial muscles, heart, and even our intestines. European Air would be the motor control, connecting many different countries (motor cortex areas) with a large international hub in the cerebellum. Each airport (structure within the brain) has preferred airlines (brain-mediated action types such as taste, vision, and motor control). But the entire brain works as many structures and neural networks (flights) work in a coordinated fashion to move information in a timely and purposeful manner.

With the understanding that I'm deviating a bit from true neurology, we can think of the memory centers (e.g. hippocampus) as the customs department. As the planes travel about, many of them must get a passport stamp of "safe" or "unsafe." When information is coded (passport stamped) as unsafe, the security personnel (amygdala) need to open up the bags and gather a bit more information. They may write up a report that is stored in your memory center. Or they may code that unsafe memory as a "do not fly" or flagged list, thus signaling a change in the way you fly (or perceive the same sensations that are being flagged) in the future. When memories are flagged, such as the "do not fly" list, we may shut down and dissociate upon our next experience to truly not even feel them again. Or they are coded with neurochemistry that flags them as such danger we become aggressive when exposed to those same sensations without even really understanding in the moment why we are experiencing them. With repeated exposure, as is often the case with adversity, the neurons themselves carry these "labels" as our neurochemistry changes how we perceive future events. When these labels change our neurochemistry, it is truly not a conscious choice as to how we respond to them in the first moments. We must rehabilitate the person without shaming them for their initial reactions and work together with them to build new experiences which recode the sensations as safe. We must change the neurochemistry to get them through customs again with "smooth sailing." I chose "smooth sailing" because sometimes the way to achieve this is by forming completely new experiences. If they can't fly, we might need to take a boat to get to our destination. For example, if an individual associates a certain body type as a threat, we may need to ensure primary caregivers are of a different body type for a while. Or if an audible alarm is terrifying to them, we need to advocate and ask school personnel to excuse them from the fire alarm drills. If a shower causes them alarm, they may need to take baths or be able to leave the door open. If a person was the instigator of their trauma, we may need to help them form relationships with animals as we work to regain their trust.

As we consider dysfunction, if a brain structure/hub is damaged, there is still hope for rehabilitation. We still have private pilots using the smaller airfields to land the information. But this will take more time and energy, and be less efficient. We can see how focusing on rehabilitating the "hubs" will give us a bigger bang for our buck. Larger airports will have larger impacts. So sometimes it benefits the therapist to work in those areas first. Dr. Perry teaches about five sequentially ordered areas of brain development: the brainstem, diencephalon, limbic system, cortex, and prefrontal cortex (Perry & Winfrey, 2021). These five brain areas are similar to continents in our air traffic metaphor. Most jets need to stop and refuel before they make it all the way around the world (from the brainstem to the cortex). If the supplies can't fly out of the brainstem (rhythm and coordination hubs), we will lack the resources and skills needed for our cortex (our reasoning and inhibition hubs). If we do not first calm the alert systems and feel as though we have the skills and capacity, we will never be able to understand the more thoughtful experiences of being in community with others and understanding societal norms and altruistic actions. If we don't feel as though we are personally safe, *at that very moment*, we can only consider treatment goals that are working to immediately decrease the stress response. Trying to target anything else in the moment will be pointless.

We must rehab the brainstem/autonomic/earliest-developing parts of the brain in order to have the foundation to rehab the later-developing, more cortical/thought-based areas. We must be able to sleep and feel safe before we think and plan. We also must consider how different parts of our brain are activated. Some portions are always on, such as our suck/swallow/breathe. These are the international airports that never close. These flights are picking up information from all over the body on a constant basis and are crucial for survival. When these brain structures/major airports have delays, the effects are experienced globally. When you are choking on a piece of food, your attention is solely on being able to breathe and swallow effectively to clear your airway. You can't take on any new foods or possibly even communicate your choking to another person in the moment when your suck/swallow/breathe rhythm is off. Side note: this is why practicing prior to the event is so important. When you practice the hand signals for choking when your cortical brain is in full-function mode, you will have a better capacity to recall this lifesaving action when you need it when the cortex is dialed down. This is an example of how practiced repetitive neural activation when we are calm can provide scaffolding for when we experience stress.

The parts of the brain that mediate survival functions are mostly automatic and will influence other parts of our brain. They take precedence when brain functional capacity is stressed. While the smaller airports can continue to work with the smaller planes, eventually they will not be able to survive without the larger hubs bringing in the resources and supplies needed to keep them going. They will quickly fatigue, and the staffing will become too stretched. When the stress becomes chronic or overwhelming, those little side airports begin to shut down. When adversity is experienced early in development, the larger hubs which regulate our emotions and attachment to our caregivers are impacted. Without strong side airports of relational buffering and co-regulation, these children have more difficulty with many other aspects of their daily activity functioning.

However, our brain hubs are designed to be able to function for a limited time in short bursts. We are able to maintain some cognitive function if a stressor is very quick and not extreme. Revisiting Dr. Perry's teachings on resilience—the ability to return to our functional baseline—is more likely when there is a relational co-regulator and the stress is patterned (it has defined or repeated expectations), predictable (we know when it will begin and end), and only mild to moderate (not severe) or for short durations. So much of our stress response is dependent upon intensity and our capacity to share the fallout with those we trust in our community. An example could be the death of a loved one. When the death is predictable, such as terminal illness or aging, and the family has a sense of community and support, the grieving process doesn't limit daily function after a few weeks. But when the death is sudden or the family does not feel supported, the grieving process can last long enough to increase the risk of vulnerability and limits to daily function. This is evidence for why care calendars for meals, checking in on grieving loved ones, and encouraging connection and perceived control can be helpful in times of grief.

As I considered activities for the KALMAR app, I used activity analysis to determine which parts of the brain "light up" with each activity. Does the activity target more than one remediation goal? For example, let's say the goal is to provide rhythmic, repetitive, relational activity to calm the brainstem and also increase a frustration tolerance for being in the presence of others. If we sit in the presence of a dog or cat, we are increasing our tolerance for being in the presence of others. But we aren't really engaging the brainstem. But if we pet or groom the dog or cat, we are now engaging both the social airports in the limbic system as well as the repetitive calming hub in the brainstem.

Going for a walk alone is a nice rhythmic, repetitive, relevant activity that stimulates the brainstem hub. But we aren't really helping to add tolerance for the presence of another being in the relational limbic system. If we add another person or a dog to our walk, we are adding a relationship to the powerful regulation equation. Sometimes, simply changing an activity ever so slightly will give it a more therapeutic "heft" as we look towards activity suggestions. I'm wondering what parts of the brain are being activated with the activity I'm doing. When I can, I try to imagine what I can bring to the therapy session to create visual fireworks on that fMRI scan. How can I send lots of planes into those hubs without overwhelming the person and causing air traffic delays? Conversely, when do I need to recognize that my client is in a personal lightning storm, and I need to shut down a few airports for them due to weather? If my client was in detention at school before the caregiver picked them up to bring them to therapy, I know to decrease the activity of the executive functioning private airfields while guiding them to land their heavy and overloaded planes by providing them with extra landing gear (increased rhythmic proprioception) and increasing the lights on the runway (less verbal and more visual commands) to guide them right where they need to be. I'm the air traffic control rerouting them to the best option given the "stormy weather." I need to bring my relational self to the room and work alongside them to get those planes landed while I give time for that storm to pass.

Our human bodies are highly dependent on developmental sequences, from the cellular level all the way up to cognitive and motor functions. We must be able to make intentional noises before we can combine them into sounds of language and eventually add context and meaning to them to engage in reciprocal dialogue. We must strengthen our abdomen by rolling over before we can learn to sequence our legs and arms to crawl, and then combine that core stability with balance and leg sequence to be able to walk and then eventually run. As we look to rehabilitate clients through an occupational therapy framework, we must be mindful of these developmental sequences that begin in the brainstem and work their way up to the cortex while simultaneously sending out private plane connections between so many different brain regions.

"Neurons that fire together, wire together"—neuropsychologist Donald Hebb first used this phrase in 1949 to describe how pathways in the brain are formed and reinforced through repetition (Mateos & Rodríguez, 2021). Another helpful metaphor as we look at brain function is to consider a spider web. A spider web is made with a thin web material. This is what the neural connections in our brain could be compared to after one connected action. As that action is repeated, that web material begins to look more like a sturdier quilting thread. After several more repetitions, the web may be formed out of yarn. As more repetitions activate the same brain structures, linking them together in that web, the yarn turns to rope and eventually a steel cable. If an action is not practiced, the web can be easily brushed away. But once an action is repeated enough, whether adaptive or not based on societal norms, it becomes difficult to change the neural bias to repeat the outcome. This is why old habits are hard to break and new habits need a lot of intentional repetition. Some factors, such as intense emotions or the influence of our proprioceptive receptors, can help with breaking down the steel cable or moving from the thread to rope more quickly. As an occupational therapist, this is an important concept to remember because it encourages us to use energetic, repetitive, and proprioceptive activities in our therapeutic treatment plans.

CHAPTER 3

The Brainstem

Tracy Stackhouse teaches that the brainstem is the first source of "embodied" experience (Weber, Whiting, Erickson, & Stackhouse, 2023). The neural tube forms three weeks after conception and divides into the brain and spinal cord. Structurally, the brainstem connects our brain to our spinal cord, literally forming the brain–body connection. It receives information from the body for the purpose of fine-tuning the regulatory functions, many of which we are not consciously aware of. It is the volume control of our life's playlist. It can "dial up" or "dial down" the volume of the current life song (state-dependent moment) being played, based on the current mental state that is being filtered through a lens of felt-safety. It "dials up" and "dials down" brain region activations to create a composition that perfectly matches that specific moment to keep us safe. Classically, we think of regulation of breath, heart rate, and balance among the primary functions of the brainstem. However, the signals that can be considered primarily sensory modulation in nature are also influencing the dialing up and dialing down of thresholds and activity across the entire nervous system, not just in the brainstem. The brainstem is simply where these coded sensations first enter and create subconscious reactions that influence our sensory integrative processing.

In our air traffic analogy, the brainstem is the largest international airport, where life ceases if it ever shuts down. It is the first anatomical brain structure to bring in and "land" new sensations. So many flights are going in and out of the brainstem, with passengers (sensory information) switching planes and making unique connections. One of the connections to another major hub airport would be the reticular activating system, which begins within the brainstem and hypothalamus and then connects forward into the cortex. This reticular activating system impacts our "A" arousal systems. Tracy Stackhouse is an occupational therapist who has some excellent resources on clinical reasoning and a deep understanding of sensory integrative processing. One of my most recommended podcasts to other therapists is her SpIRiTed Conversations, which she hosts with Australian pediatric occupational therapists Michelle Maunder and Cory Dundon (Stackhouse, MacInnes, & Maunder, n.d.). I highly recommend her work for those wanting to know more about her models and the arousal system. In her podcast, she talks about "A" functions of **A**utonomic arousal, central nervous system (CNS) **A**rousal, **A**ffect, **A**ction, and **A**ttention, and how they influence our mental states and functional capacity. Tracy gives language to how these processes further illustrate the interconnectedness of our brain "hubs" as they relate to function. **Autonomic arousal** in the brainstem interacts with the diencephalon to create a just-right state of alert in regard to the sensation and the signal of safety or threat. Sensation also contributes to general **CNS arousal** and the level of general activation or rest across the whole nervous system. **Affect** interacts with the limbic functions to help us respond emotionally. **Action** interacts with the cortical and cerebellar areas involved with the motor systems to move our bodies in response to the sensation. **Attention** interacts with the activation of focal energies across the brain and with the prefrontal cortex areas to help us know how to assess, attend to, and store memories, and reflect on the sensation. Thinking about these "A" functions gives us a clear example of how the brainstem is a connecting hub that influences every aspect of our functionality. Just as we use Dr. Perry's arousal continuum as a lens for our clinical reasoning with activity selection, we use Tracy's "A" functions to help us use activity analysis to determine which "A" or combination of "As" the client is having difficulty with in that state-dependent moment.

To survive, we have to be able to feel our bodies in relation to our environment and, in particular, in relation to our carers who are our comforters and co-regulators. We have to be able to feel pain and comfort not just from a modulation, "is it safe?" perspective, but also from a discriminative perspective that provides us with the details of the sensation. Thus, our modulation and discrimination functions lay the foundation for our neuroception and our perception, which helps to inform our experience of what is happening to us and what the resultant responses feel like. This all creates the felt container of our experience.

"Seeking" or "avoiding" is common phraseology in some OT approaches, even mine as a seasoned therapist until my understanding deepened. But seeking and avoiding isn't an accurate way to describe this process. Seeking or avoiding describes a choice or preference, when the action is actually a subconscious biological result of our neurological interpretation of the sensation. When we look at the work of Dr. Stephen Porges and his polyvagal theory, we can see that more accurate verbiage comes from an understanding that the information from our sensory modulation system tells us to move *towards safety* or *away from threat* as the first tier of response within the brainstem (Porges, 2011). Our second-tier responses in the higher cortical structures then form the thoughtful actions and preferences related to our sensations once we attain a perceived state of felt-safety. Within this seeking felt-safety, we may move more *actively* or *passively* towards safety. We may become hypervigilant or aggressive if we feel as though we can physically and actively change the proximity of the threat. An example would be running away from or throwing a chair at a carer who is perceived as harming us. Or we may dissociate by avoiding social gatherings or staying in bed when a situation seems too threatening to our nervous system.

Sometimes safety is moving towards what is familiar (even if it is a threat), because our brain is wired to give more attention and use more energy towards unknown things whereas familiarity is often coded as safety in our neuroreceptors (Porges, 2011). An example is when someone stays in an abusive relationship because they fear the unknown of being alone would be worse than being abused. Another example is when a person initiates a physical fight that they believe is imminent. A child may even run away from a loving foster home or become upset with holiday giftings because it is too unfamiliar from their past experiences with gift-giving holidays. This reaction to sensory stimulation is also dependent on what our basic regulatory capacity is with our arousal, affect, attention, and action networks. Our capacity to change our response is influenced if we are cold, hungry, have an autoimmune response from illness (autonomic arousal), feel depressed, scared, or joyful (affect), if we are distracted by something interesting or frightening (attention), or if our muscles and motor pathways are working efficiently (action).

First and foremost for our regulatory capacity is our sense of connection, attachment, and co-regulation. While these may seem to be higher-order social and emotional processes, the capacity to connect is processed at *every* level of our nervous system—beginning in the brainstem. The brainstem is essential to all our general regulatory capacities.

As we look at activities that rehabilitate the brainstem, we recognize that there are many things mediated in this area that are not discussed in this book. For a more thorough understanding of brain-based mediated functioning, it is recommended that the reader explore Dr. Perry's NMT™ metric by visiting www.neurosequential.com/NMT. Our goal for this book is to focus on OT-relevant areas of functioning that are in the 2022 version of the NMT™ (Perry, 2013). Some of the assessed areas are mediated in multiple portions of the brain, such as "eating." The suck, swallow, breathe sequence originates in the brainstem. Food choices, preferences, and tongue control originate in other cortical places, and these functions interconnect, like the air traffic analogy discussed earlier. "Difficulty with food" is listed under the brainstem because brainstem-mediated tasks are considered first for intervention in the Neurosequential Model. If the individual can't suck/swallow/breathe from the brainstem function, their food preferences (not wanting to eat specific veggies or proteins) simply won't be a factor in treatment until the food can be swallowed without fear of choking. It is best practice to start with the lowest-mediated, foundational portions of the brain. For this book, I will be using some generalizations in our categorization with the end goal of helping the reader look at human functioning through activity analysis with a brain-based lens. It brings value to our treatment sessions when we look at food as one of the first therapeutic goals because nutrition and the ability to eat a variety of foods directly impacts many areas of human functioning.

With generalizations acknowledged, we begin our NMT™-inspired activity analysis for some of the categorical functions found in Dr. Perry's NMT™ metric:

- difficulty with food

- heart rate normalization

- temperature regulation

- breathing

- weight as it relates to nutrition intake

- autoimmune issues such allergies, eczema, and bowel issues

- muscular movement of the eyes.

Difficulty with Food

I like the analogy that it is non-productive to paint walls when the drywall behind them is crumbling. When a child struggles with food, they often struggle with many other daily activities. Much social etiquette and manners involve food, as it is deeply steeped in relationships. When a person struggles with oral motor control, food refusal, or sensory overwhelm related to mealtimes, they often struggle with societal norms, being labeled as resistive or sloppy and given punitive consequences for behaviors that are not in their capacity to remedy. Spending hours *telling* someone they need to eat better is very unlikely to actually help them succeed. We need to use our activity analysis skills to better understand *why* they aren't eating well.

When giving therapeutic activity recommendations for food, the activity may benefit other functions as well. If a child has a high heart rate and doesn't eat well, I begin to wonder if working on breath would be beneficial. Breath is something that influences both heart rate and the suck/swallow/breathe sequence required for knowing when to chew, take a breath, and swallow.

As we investigate difficulty with food, let's consider a case study.

J only eats white and yellow foods. His plate is full of rice, French fries, chicken nuggets, bread, and macaroni and cheese. These are foods he will tolerate, but he still doesn't eat them. If Mom changes anything, he might refuse to eat for the next two meals or more. Because he doesn't eat well during the day, he often wakes up hungry at night. His growling tummy prevents him from falling asleep. He gets frequent tummy aches because the excessive amount of cheese in his diet makes him constipated. With this constipation, even moving around can be painful for him, so he becomes very sedentary and does not get much exercise. Yet he is perceived as overweight. How can a child who eats so little be overweight?

While this one case study could go 1000 different directions, how do we even know where to start? If we use the NMT™ lens, we start at the beginning. We go back developmentally as far as we can in physical, oral motor, and brain development. What was this child's birth experience like? The rhythm of the human suck/swallow/breathe is developed within the womb. In premature infants, we find that they are able to suck and swallow at around 25–28 weeks' gestation. It isn't until around 32 weeks' gestation that their lungs can support the breathing function. It takes thousands of repetitions to develop that skill. What was the mother's hormonal experience during that last trimester? Was her system flooded with increased heart rate or stress hormones that somehow influenced the development of this rhythm? When my heart is beating rapidly, it sends a signal to my brain to take quick, shallow breaths to keep my blood oxygenated. The number of breaths per minute will then influence my suck/swallow/breathe sequence. If I'm breathing too fast, I will feel as though I need to inhale when a bite is taken and then I feel at risk of choking.

I've heard horrific stories of abuse involving the mouth. Stories of parents who place hot sauce on their child's tongue as a punishment for not eating or a mother who poured hot oil into her child's mouth during a hallucination episode. All of these will develop strong associations with negative experiences when food is put close to the mouth. Because of this, we focus on safety first and foremost when dealing with food. If we can't *trust* the food or the person feeding us, we will not be able to tolerate any type of food exploration. We playfully engage the mouth. We may even start with non-food items such as bubbles, lip gloss, or face paint.

In order to work therapeutically with food, we must also address the emotional associations surrounding food. Food *feels* good. Infants eat many times a day. Biologically, those are times when we are connected skin to skin and eye to eye with our mothers, sharing in oxytocin and other bonding chemicals. It is through food that we are biologically wired to form our first attachments. Caregivers quickly realize that providing food is one of the quickest ways to calm a baby. When something happens to hinder this process (cleft palate, tied tongue, reflux), there is often shame and feelings of inadequacy and helplessness from the caregiver. They are not able to meet the basic needs of the infant, and there are countless reminders throughout the day of this struggle. In an effort of self-preservation, the caregiver may pull away from the infant, further hindering this attachment process. Modern society has created many clever and creative ways to feed a newborn and infant. We use nursing blankets in public that decrease that eye contact. We prop bottles up in the crib that lead to ear infections from poor head placement while eating. With a propped-up bottle, the child does not get the repetitive neural feedback that his needs are met through the response of his caregiver. Because of this, we must now consider how this has impacted the attachment and social consequences of this more disconnected approach, especially when there is neglect and early childhood adversity.

Once we establish safety and trust, we need to actually look at breathing rates and if the child can safely swallow while coordinating their open airway. If you have ever choked on a particular food, you may easily understand how easy it is to reject a food that threatens your basic life survival skill of breathing. We rehabilitate the suck/swallow/breathe through blowing activities, strengthening breath support through diaphragm exercises, or changing the food consistency. (Soft and smooth foods like yogurt, banana, and avocado are easiest to swallow quickly and efficiently.) For repeated success to disarm the fear of choking, we need to assess how the food is managed within the mouth. Does the child have adequate tongue movement to clear the teeth and form a bolus (smooshed gathering of food that forms a "ball" as it slides down the esophagus)? Can the child tolerate the texture of the food in the mouth? Do they have the sensory awareness to understand where it is motorically and if they enjoy the taste or texture as a personal experience? Can they handle the complex textures of foods that are different consistencies? If we think back to the white and yellow food diet in our case study, we can see how foods that are high in fat and carbohydrates tend to require very little saliva and tongue movement to get them ready to swallow. There is little effort required for that food to feel *safe* in our mouth. For some of the children I work with, more sensory information is required for the child to *feel* the sensation of the food. For these children, salty, spicy, crunchy foods sometimes give them enough input to signal the muscles in the mouth to know how to handle the food.

Food is such a complex issue that involves in utero rhythms, motor planning that is heavily reliant upon early social and emotional care taking, and independent felt experiences surrounding the feeding experiences. It is also incredibly multisensory. Our food preferences are highly dependent upon our familiarity (heritage) and the personal and unique ways we interpret how it looks, feels, tastes, smells, and even sounds. Sound could be the crack of bread as it is broken, or the way crunchy things sound as they echo within the oral cavity. We even hear the sound of popcorn popping as we anticipate a family movie night as we salivate with the smell of the butter melting.

Once we have considered some of the *why* behind the food patterns, activity analysis helps me identify how I can adapt or modify the experience to help my clients be more successful with food.

First, I must consider the phrase a colleague, Nikki Nootboom, once said to me: "Heal the parent to heal the child." Dr. Perry emphasizes that if we are to be able to engage a person in the relational, repetitive, rhythmic healing activities, we must first make sure that the adult caregiver responsible for providing these experiences has the capacity within themselves to do so. With food, there is much rejection and self-shame upon the caregiver. If an experience that is played out and practiced a minimum of three times per day is not positive, I need to work with the caregiver to reframe the "behavior" and create self-compassion and motivation to continue to engage and be a positive influence for these interactions. When the caregiver is constantly bracing themselves for the refusal of the food, their body language will signal disconnect to the child and further inhibit the desired attachment necessary for successful food remediation. Conversely, when food is the source of comfort, the caregiver must also recognize ways in which they can help shift the desire for connection from food to people. The key to this shift may lie in consistency. So often, I work with caregivers who have "tried everything." They have tried so many diets and so many gimmicks. They simply lose the stamina to be consistent and predictable. But the human body craves routine and predictability. I once saw something that really resonated with me. It was a meme with a grid containing several blueberries and a goldfish cracker. Under each blueberry, there was a descriptor word such as "sweet," "tart," "squishy," and "firm." Under the cracker were the words "The same. Every. Single. Time." This graphic really stuck with me – how many of our "target foods" such as fruits, vegetables, and even meats can change in regard to sensory experience. Yet highly processed foods, the ones my clients tolerate, are incredibly predictable. For so many people I work with, their lives began with unpredictability and chaos. Their precious little brains were grasping for "normal," for consistency, for predictability. For many of them, this grasping created strong physical, developmental, and emotional habits that involve highly processed and consistent food.

As we think back to J in our case study, we first work with Mom and validate her feelings. We may see feelings of failure, shame, and purposeful rejections. We can understand that even when she is trying her best, she is exhausted, and so many things she has tried have failed. She can't take the risk of trying something new, because if it doesn't work on the first try, she's worried he will slip into more rigidity and spiral out of control quickly, and she will have failed at a basic survival skill for her son. After we validate her feelings, we can help her understand the root of these behaviors that are leading to both the rejection of the foods and her felt-sense of the rejection of her love. We can help her understand that it has more to do with J's sensational interpretation of the events and less with her presentation and involvement with them. We can help her understand that "Of course, you get angry and sometimes yell or demonstrate anger or withdrawal with food refusal. That is horribly personal and frustrating." But when you know better, you do better. Once we can identify that Mom's feelings are understandable and *human*, we can help her find the brief capacity to pause before her emotional reactions overtake the moment. We can gain compassion for how difficult it must be to have such a complicated relationship with food. I once read in a blog how we can have empathy. The writing was about a mother's struggle to be in the car with her seemingly ungrateful and entitled teenager. As she truly listened to her teen's emotion behind her complaints, she realized it is more difficult in this moment to *be* someone who is struggling than it is to *be with* someone who is struggling. In our case study, this empathy buys us the time for a deep exhale breath for Mom. Of note, it is the *exhale* breath that moves us towards calm and the *inhale* breath that moves us towards alert. We encourage her to keep her tone of voice kind and release some of the pressure that is pushing J into further control and resistance as he grasps to find safety and trust in the moment.

Next, we become curious activity analysis detectives. Can we increase J's heart rate prior to eating with some quick jumping jacks? Can we decrease his heart rate prior to eating by blowing a feather across the table or making a bubble cone in his chocolate (protein powder) shake? Do either of these activities seem to have any effect on his food tolerance? What about changing the seating? Can he swallow more easily when he is standing next to the table? What about sitting on a therapy ball? Does he need more or less movement? What about allowing him to sit at a different seat at the table? Does the head of the table empower him so that he is in more control? Do the arms of that head chair provide him with more postural stability to sit up tall, which opens up the ribcage a bit and provides support for his diaphragm and ribcage, stabilized through his shoulders now that his arms are braced? Is he less likely to be distracted by what is outside the window? Or does the welcoming light shining through the panes constrict his pupils and help him focus on the bright, welcoming food on his plate? Would eating by candlelight change the overall mood of his visual eating experience? How can we change the physical environment that has nothing to do with actual food on the plate?

Once we have explored the external environment, we can begin to look at the food itself and how it relates to his oral motor skills. Are the foods a good match for him in consistency? Does he have enough saliva to soften the dryer foods? Do mushy foods mix with his saliva and become too wet? Is the food so thin it feels as if it is going to run into his trachea/windpipe? Are the textures so complex that it's difficult to understand where things are in his mouth in order to be able to easily form the bolus? Are his jaw and cheek muscles strong enough to handle the repetitions needed to safely masticate (chew) the food adequately? Think of how long a tough piece of meat or a carrot needs to be chewed compared to a soft cracker. What about the firmness of the food? If we cook our carrots, they require less muscle work to chew them.

What about smell and sound? How does cooking affect this? Things that are steaming from warmth will reach the smell receptors in the nose more quickly and easily. They may be softer, but the smell has now been amplified. Freezing food decreases the smell but increases the hardness of the texture. Do either of these modifications help J?

As we ask these questions, we can be mindful of how long this process can take. For many of the children we work with, change is incredibly difficult. Most people would prefer a known experience that is negative over an unknown experience that is positive. We crave routine. So we can't change too many things at once. It might also take several exposures before we know if something can be tolerated. I once read that a child needs a minimum of 12 exposures to a food before they will even consider it. Having the patience to calmly present nutritious food that feels like life or death 12 times requires a lot of outside support for the caregiver.

As J begins to feel some predictability and safety surrounding an understanding that his food rejection is not as personal as it feels, there is hope that he may eventually find help for the possible complex reasons he has limited food preferences. Very seldom is it purely an oral motor weakness, postural instability, or trauma association. Because eating is heavily influenced within early development and brainstem function, it is often a multifaceted treatment approach. Hopefully, this section has given the reader a bit of insight into this particular type of case.

When assessing food difficulty, I look at oral motor skills, variety of food intake, and patterns in food tolerance or rejection. I look at a variety of food in regard to nutrition and sensory characteristics such as taste, texture, and smell. I consider body mass compared to caloric intake and refer to feeding specialists when I don't see improvements.

Suggestions for therapeutic activities that help with **difficulty with food** taken from the KALMAR app:

- **Allow child control** of food choices and encourage participation in meal prep. When a child has difficulty understanding the sensory input of food to adequately chew and swallow, it can be helpful for them to know exactly what is in their food. The predictive element of making their own food can work wonders to disarm a fear of the unknown.

- **Consider medication side effects** and their impact on appetite. When requesting someone with poor motor planning take a pill, it is helpful to request that they tilt their chin forward (towards belly) when swallowing.

- **Consider modifications** to food presentation. Since cold food releases less olfactory steam, it may be better tolerated. Cold food also has increased temperature sensory input. Slicing carrots lengthwise makes them easier to chew than slicing them as discs because of the matched anatomical orientation to the molars. Cooked broccoli smooshes together in the mouth while raw broccoli tends to scatter and spread, getting lost in the gums. When a food is rejected, work with the client to see if there are simple ways to change how we prepare it that could help them tolerate the food better.

- **Give extra grace** surrounding nutrition. For many clients, food is presented at least three times per day in unpleasant circumstances. At least three times per day there is conflict surrounding food. As much as possible, try to make food less of a power struggle. Lower your nutritional goals if necessary.

- **Refer** to a nutritionist, speech therapist, occupational therapist, or clinical psychologist for eating disorders. When a child is on the extreme ends of the weight charts, specialized professionals can help provide the support needed to help an individual meet their food-related goals.

Heart rate normalization

Our heart is a muscle that makes sure oxygen is circulated effectively throughout our body. When the heart stops even momentarily, that lack of oxygen circulation can lead to tissue death. When that tissue is brain tissue, the effect can be catastrophic. Your heart pumping that oxygen around to your cells is a vital survival function. It is also a basic rhythm of life. The mother's heartbeat is one of the first regulatory mechanisms for the embryo. There is a constant thump and bump against the chest wall and artery that neighbors the womb as the baby grows. Maternal heart rate will influence the baby's heart rate as they co-regulate together. The rhythmic thumping against the chest wall is one of the very first ways we co-regulate with our caregiver. It's no surprise some of the most relaxing music has a similar rhythm of 60–80 beats per minute (bpm).

When we move our skeletal muscles, the heart speeds up to make sure that this oxygen is fresh and ready to provide the energy for an athlete or fleeing person to move quickly. When we are sedentary, our heart rate slows, and our blood doesn't circulate as quickly. Like most muscles, the heart is use dependent. Heart rate and blood pressure are autonomic responses to both external and internal stimuli. With chronic stress, when an individual experiences prolonged increased heart rate, it becomes a pattern. Because of this, their base heart rate will generally be faster than someone who is not in a vigilant state of needing to be ready to escape.

When considering heart rate, I ask my clients to wear my Apple Watch or ask the caregiver to use a simple monitor to gather data on resting heart rate and average heart rate throughout daily activity. A normal heart rate for a child should be 75–110. For adults, it should be 60–80. When I see data for a child with a higher-than-normal heart rate, I begin to wonder if they are in a chronically high-alert or activated state.

This heart rate monitor data has been a valuable tool in my own sensory space. So many of my clients report that they can't feel their resting heartbeat. It is also a very subjective and non-judgmental way to show caregivers data about how their child is perceiving the world as a constant threat. I've also used it to show how some of my dissociative teens are actually very alert and not as "calm" as they appear.

As treatment progresses and this data normalizes, it gives further evidence that can be documented about how the client's internal functions are changing with treatment.

Table 3.1 Things that increase or decrease heart rate

Things that can *increase* heart rate	Things that can *decrease* heart rate
Exercise	Meditation
Sharp inhale	Slow exhale
Music with a bpm over 120	Music with a bpm under 80
Cold water	Warm/lukewarm water
Light touch	Deep pressure
Alerting thoughts	Calming thoughts
Startling environmental stimuli	Relaxing environmental stimuli
Medication	Medication

Note: As you review the activities in the KALMAR suggestion boxes, you may notice repeats. This ties back to how activities cross into multiple brain regions. Behind the scenes of the KALMAR online app is how we weight the activities based on how many of the target remediation areas they will help. For example, animal-assisted therapies can help with heart rate, temperature regulation, relationships, and even sleep. So this is repeated in several KALMAR suggestion sections. For the purpose of this book, I will keep suggestions to five per section. For a longer list of activity suggestions, please use the KALMAR tool available at kalmar.creativetherapies.com.

Suggestions for therapeutic activities that help with **heart rate normalization** taken from the KALMAR app:

- **Animal-assisted therapies.** Larger animals such as horses and big dogs tend to have lower resting heart rates that can be "contagious" to humans. Simply sitting close to these animals can influence our own pace of heartbeat. Try to find an animal that matches the energy tempo of the client. Ask the client which animal they "relate to" and pair them with that animal if possible. Chickens can match a very energetic client, while a rabbit or goat will be calmer.

A snake can be great for a highly alert but dissociative adolescent. It moves slowly but provides that alertness of, well, being a snake.

- **Deep breathing exercises.** Our lungs and heart are anatomically connected. Blood must circulate first in the lungs to absorb the oxygen that the heart then pumps to the body. The amount of oxygen in the blood is moderated and then regulated by the heart with varying heartbeat cycle speeds. Slowly inhaling more air brings in more oxygen so that the heart doesn't need to pump as fast to distribute the same volume.

- **Heart rate monitor/sport data watches for biofeedback.** While it is difficult to tell your heart a specific beat number since it is primarily mediated in the brainstem areas, we can be mindful of our breath and even our state of internal safety so that we can send "cues" to the brainstem of the state we want to be in. We can increase quick short breaths to bring it up or think of a rhythmic, relaxing location such as looking at waves on a beach or wind-blown aspen leaves in the mountains to influence the cadence of our heartbeat.

- **Meditation** is a common "top-down" activity to lower the heart rate. The goal is to have the person focus on cues of safety that will move the focus of the mind into safe calm instead of anxious fear. When the brain does not perceive threat, it does not send signals to the heart to increase blood flow to prepare for action.

- **Walking** stimulates blood flow as the muscles use the oxygen in the blood for energy to contract in sequence to move the body. The faster the muscles need to fire, the more oxygen is needed and thus the faster the heart will beat to move this oxygen to the muscles. Walking is a very rhythmic/repetitive activity that can be helpful when looking for a quiet parallel activity with a caregiver.

Temperature regulation

Temperature regulation is another brainstem response that has many connections to other areas. A common social exchange is asking about the weather. Humans are constantly engaging and talking about temperatures. Living in Texas, where weather temperatures can be extreme, being aware of the temperature is incredibly important. We can't live in extreme temperatures. Indeed, our temperature is one of the most common ways to assess illness or infection. When we have a fever, our body is fighting something. When a person has difficulty with regulating their temperature, their brainstem becomes engaged. The brainstem is wired for immediate survival.

Our brainstem works really hard to keep our body temperature regulated. The nerve receptors that interpret temperature are more sensitive to cold than to hot. It takes a larger difference to notice a change in warmer temperature than it does cooler. This is one reason a cool breeze is perceived as an alerting chill. Since temperature physically transduces from hot to cold, it is easier to remove heat and cool a body than it is to warm it up. Hence, our survival is more dependent upon feeling cool temperatures.

People who have experienced adversity sometimes perceive outside temperatures differently and they have trouble regulating their core body temperatures. Clinically, I often hear of clients who don't dress appropriately for the weather, or they are "always cold" or "always hot." Seeing weather-inappropriate clothing causes me to be curious about whether this person has a high or slow metabolism, a tactile sensation need or intolerance, or a lack of reasoning ability to know what to wear when.

Suggestions for therapeutic activities that help with **temperature regulation** taken from the KALMAR app:

- **Felt–safety.** Work with clients so that there is a "felt-sense" of safety. As much as possible, allow them control of clothing, food choices, fans, heat packs, etc. Help them get in touch with how sensations feel from their perspective.

- **Textiles.** Cooling wraps, extra clothing, and weighted blankets can influence temperature while also providing proprioceptive input. When someone has experienced trauma, it is best for them to be able to have control over the use of these items. They could react negatively to forced use of these items, especially if they were previously held down or forced to wear specific clothing items.

- **Showers** can provide a means to quickly cool or warm the body based on the water temperature.

- **Dietary interventions.** The Adverse Childhood Experiences (ACE) study discovered that people who have experienced adversity have a higher incidence of health diagnosis such as diabetes, obesity, and heart disease (Felitti *et al.*, 1998). Each of these ACE-related diagnoses come with food regulations. Our metabolism and the amount of surface area of our body will also influence our base temperature and ability to cool and heat our bodies. When someone is in a state of stress, sugary and salty food can provide an increase in dopamine, a reward hormone. People who have experienced trauma therefore may need assistance with healthy meal planning and support with dietary restrictions.

- **Movement** will increase blood flow, which will increase temperature. Rhythmic, repetitive movement also helps to "calm" the brainstem and help the person self-regulate, especially when agitated.

Breathing

The medulla is located in the brainstem and is responsible for a number of reflexive actions, including vomiting, swallowing, coughing, and sneezing. It controls our respiratory functions which bring the oxygen in to be carried through the blood cells to help us convert glucose into energy. Without oxygen from good breath regulation, we cannot sustain life.

While oxygen is mostly controlled without us thinking about it, we do have neural pathways that can have a top-down influence to increase or decrease our breath rate consciously.

Because of our conscious awareness of our breathing, "just breathe" or "take a breath" can be well-intended suggested strategies to help a person. However, it is rarely effective when the person is in a high-alert state. When a person is in a high-alert state, it is difficult to access those frontal top-down structures to relay that "calm down" information. When someone is in distress, a common response is to gasp for breath or take a sharp, deep inhale as the body prepares itself to have the energy it needs to fight or flee. The inhale preps the body for action while the exhale signals the body to calm. So, when someone cues you to take a breath, they are actually asking you to prepare for activation. Instead, I have more success when I help put a person in a diaphragm-supported position such as sitting up tall (not tilting the head back or collapsing the abdomen). I then model a breath with them where I emphasize the out-breath. While a pulse oximeter can be helpful to know if someone has lowered amounts of oxygen in their blood, I seldom use one clinically because it is most beneficial in a hospital or rehab setting when oxygen needs administering for critically low levels. For most people, there are other indications of being short of breath without being in the critical zone such as labored breathing, lethargy, and slumped posture. I even see eating abnormalities related to breath, such as gulping food or refusing complex textures.

When someone doesn't have good core support or diaphragm control, it can hinder oxygen capacity. I have my clients put their bodies in different positions and take breaths when they are calm. I help them to notice how leaning too far forward compresses the diaphragm to limit the amount of air they can bring in. We put our pinky in our belly buttons and watch our hand move to distinguish between belly breathing, which is used for long breath support, and upper chest/upper lobe breathing, which is more activating for those quick but small oxygen bursts. We also talk about how sometimes food can influence our breathing as the cerebellum begins to coordinate our suck/swallow/breathe patterns. Food that is easier to swallow appears safer for someone whose suck/swallow/breathe rhythm is impaired.

Oxygen levels are influenced by sleep, exercise, even our altitude and environmental humidity levels. Casinos in Las Vegas long ago discovered that if they eliminate natural light and pump in extra oxygen to the gaming floor, people will stay alert longer and spend more money because their natural biorhythms will be influenced and the oxygen will make them less sleepy. Some people experience sleep apnea where they have difficulty with regulating their breathing patterns when they fall asleep. When we exercise, we improve our lung capacity to be more efficient. If we live in a highly polluted area, the air we breathe will have more pollutants and could cause damage to our lungs and lower our intake capacity. This is especially impactful for people who are living in crowded areas with poor air quality. Cool air is less dense, and the higher in altitude you go, the thinner the air gets. Even the smells in our environment can influence our oxygen levels. Pleasant smells encourage a slow inhale to savor that sensory experience and absorb the oxygen, while an unpleasant smell tends to cause breathing to be quicker in both inhalation and exhalation.

When I have a client who seems lethargic, has chronic allergies, or gives an indication that they are having trouble breathing, I work on this as one of my first goals. So much is dependent upon good breath support.

Suggestions for therapeutic activities that help with **breathing** taken from the KALMAR app:

- **Animal-assisted therapies.** When someone is hurt by a person, it can be difficult for another person to be trusted. Animals have a way of quickly establishing felt-safety for many of my clients. With most animals, we can also see their breath rate. When my clients can see and even sometimes feel the animal's breath, we can then discuss their own breath. Many people I work with tend to hold their breath or take shallow breaths. Drawing attention to the animal's breath is a non-shaming way to help people who have experienced trauma draw attention to their own breath.

- **Meditation, yoga, pilates,** and other rhythmic movement activities influence the breath. When we have good guided practices, our focus is often brought to our breath.

- **Oral motor activities.** Our breath support begins with a strong diaphragm muscle. To exercise this muscle, many OTs use oral motor activities such as blowing feathers, "hot soup," bubbles (both in soap as well as through a wand), and balloons. Smelling pleasant things can facilitate deep breathing exercises.

- **A fan** blowing air over the face can encourage a person to inhale.

Bouncing on a large therapy ball in a seated position pushes air up through the diaphragm and also encourages breath support as well as vocalization as air moves up through the vocal cords.

- **Core-strengthening exercises.** Cardiovascular exercises can increase the blood flow that will facilitate the need for more oxygen. But without a good core support, the lungs will be restricted and unable to draw in a full, oxygenizing breath.

- **Drinking thicker liquids from a straw** puts liquid further back so not as much tongue coordination is required to swallow. This can be helpful for someone who experienced neglect and did not go through the developmental stages of drinking from a nipple (bottle or breast) first and then slowly learning to move the tongue around to place food in an optimal position for easy swallowing. Food may have been scarce and eating forced or quick so that the child becomes fearful of choking. If they do not have good breath support and strong suck/swallow/breathe coordination arising from the brainstem, straws are an excellent way to help this child get adequate nutrition.

Weight as it relates to nutrition intake

When the human body is in a state of high alert, digestion is not a brain hierarchy priority. When the blood is being pumped into the muscles to make fight and flight easier, the gut is left with little energy to digest and absorb efficiently. Because of this, stress can influence our bowel function, weight, and nutrition intake. Stress can cause cravings for salty or fatty food or decrease the appetite. It can lead to poor sleep, which can then lead to a desire to eat energy-increasing high-carbohydrate foods. Metabolism is dependent upon regular intervals of eating. When food is sporadically available, our metabolism will work to maximize the caloric availability. I've had many clients who decrease their food intake and yet their body weight does not reflect the low caloric intake. Our bodies are fascinating structures that are designed to keep us alive. The body will hold on to fat storage if it feels it will be starved anytime soon. Or it will shed weight quickly when preparing itself to be able to flee quickly. Because of this, nutrition is highly associated with trauma.

People who experience trauma may be on medications that have appetite side effects. When a child is in hypervigilance and moves a lot, they burn a lot of calories. People who have experienced neglect may also have difficulty identifying hunger sensations. Thus, they may have poor dietary intake routines. So many social events and rituals involve food as a way to show acceptance and care for one another. Food is tied to social acceptance and physically meeting the needs of others. When a person lacks social connections and feelings of worth, they may look to food as something they can control or use as a reward to boost feel-good dopamine hormone levels. Foods that have high contents of sugars, salts, and fats tend to provide the highest dopamine surges. I find it interesting to think about this as I think about foods such as chips, cakes, and cocktails, and how we often pair them with social connections and gathering places like bars and parties. Nutritious food is also typically more expensive than highly processed food that has a longer shelf life and is easier to store and prepare.

Food is a very complex issue for many people who have experienced adversity. Because of this, there are many reasons that there may be discrepancies relating to nutrition intake. When nutrition is a goal my clients want to work on, I very carefully, non-judgmentally, and compassionately get curious about the food they eat. I listen for dietary restrictions or preferences. Sometimes, a simple offer of coffee will open the door to very insightful food conversations where I might learn that my client only eats certain foods. Maybe they only eat at certain times. I have several children on my caseload currently who try to hoard snacks and are in fear of not having food later. Sometimes, the reported caloric intake doesn't match what I see physically. For people who experienced early trauma or adversity, their clothing size is often incongruent with the number of calories, carbs, fats, or proteins they consume. Often, I have clients report that they eat very few meals and yet struggle with a seemingly low metabolism. Other times, I have clients whose caregivers report are eating "sooooo much" and yet I can still easily see their ribs. When this is the case, I try to offer support for nutritional counseling, oral motor skills, and social aspects of connected and non-judgmental food habits. When needed, I refer to a counselor who specializes in eating issues, a nutrition specialist, or speech therapist to assist me.

Suggestions for therapeutic activities that help with **weight as it relates to nutrition** taken from the KALMAR app:

- **Choice.** Allow the client to choose where to sit, what music to play in the background, or how intense the lighting should be during meals. This helps to give the person a sense of control. It also is a tangible way to let them know you care about their preferences and respect them.

- **Nutrition apps** such as FitnessPal can be a non-judgmental and very objective way to notice nutrition habits. Protein-rich foods, vitamins, and supplements can all be charted and encouraged through the use of a nutrition app.

- **Refer** to a clinical psychologist for eating disorders.

- **Special reflux pillows** can be helpful if a person has reflux. When our stomach is "upset" from stress, it might produce acidic secretions that find their way up the throat.

- **Eat meals together** without stress. People who experience trauma, adversity, or chronic stress might turn to food for comfort or avoid it due to physical nausea from the body's response to the stress. Increasing the mealtime stress by counting calories or demanding they eat certain portions can feed into a stressful food loop where they get even more avoidant or pursuant. Making mealtime about connection and engagement rather than calories and control can go a long way towards encouraging healthy eating habits.

Autoimmune issues such allergies, eczema, and bowel issues

Autoimmune issues include seasonal allergies, food allergies, bumps on the skin, and frequent diarrhea or constipation. Clinically, I see children with purple rings under the eyes or a persistent postnasal cough or runny nose. Constant clearing of the throat is another symptom. The brainstem mediates the consistency and frequency of the bowels, so "inability to potty train" likely involves other higher cortical areas if there is not a medical diagnosis.

I loved reading Dr. Bessel van der Kolk's book *The Body Keeps the Score* (2014). I highlighted and nodded along with all the things I see in my clinical practice. So many of my clients had physical symptoms of psychological distress. While it has limitations on sample size and wasn't intended to be a "one and done," the ACEs study does highlight how so many people who experience adversity have body-related diagnoses. When we consider allergies and eczema, we can view them as the body's desire to get rid of toxins. It seems that when we are trying to remove emotional toxins, our physical systems go into overdrive to remove the physical toxins and our immune responses go into overdrive. When we have limitations on diets due to diabetes or allergies, we are also limiting nutritional intake and may be lacking essential vitamins and minerals if we can't afford supplements.

Stress plays a direct role in our bowels. When we are stressed, we aren't relaxed enough to void. In my clinic, some of my clients pass gas as they relax in the Lycra, a stretchy and supportive material often used in therapeutic activities. I often tell the caregivers that I'm not at all embarrassed or concerned. Rather, I'm thrilled! Passing gas is a nice indication to me that my client is starting to relax the rectal sphincter muscle, which tells me his other muscles are probably relaxing as well. Passing gas in Miss Marti's room is something to be celebrated and often giggled about as we lean into the connection of the shared olfactory experience.

Suggestions for therapeutic activities that help with **autoimmune issues** such as allergies, eczema, and bowel issues taken from the KALMAR app:

- **Compression clothing**, such as stretchy sportswear or swim sunscreen shirts, protects the skin from the sun, which can often flare autoimmune skin issues. It also helps protect the skin from scratching and increases retained moisture.

- **Massage** can help move inflammation out of the muscles and joints where it accumulates in many autoimmune diseases. Massage also releases serotonin, which can help with pain relief.

- **Nutrition apps** such as FitnessPal can be helpful to ensure that an individual is getting adequate nutrition content when diets must be restricted because of dietary allergies. Some autoimmune diseases respond best to low-carb or non-root food diets. Nutrition apps can help ensure that dietary needs are being met with respect to the limitations.

- **Provide a sensory calm area** for the individual to self-regulate. When an individual has autoimmune issues, they often don't feel "well" and therefore can use more environmental support and adaptations to help them tolerate their sensory environment. A warm bath may soothe skin lesions or a cool bath may help to numb them. Allowing the individual voice and choice in the selection of "calming" sensations can be beneficial.

- **Rhythmic exercise** helps to give a rhythm and balance to the cerebellum and brainstem and decreases the workload of those structures through the predictability. Exercise also releases endorphins that help an individual feel better when affected by an autoimmune disease.

Muscular movement of the eyes

Some of the first muscles a baby has conscious control over are the eye muscles. Even a simple arm wave is jerky and uncoordinated in the beginning as the bones grow and tendons stretch, and proprioceptive receptors refine their efficiency. Leg muscles weeble and wobble as a toddler "toddles" while learning to walk. But the eyes develop very early on; not only are they one of the only reliably controlled muscles for an infant, but they are also their literal window onto the world. The infant bonds with the caregiver through eye contact. Much of their sensory experience is analyzed and interpreted through the eyes in the first few days and months of life. Even the vestibular system is influenced by what our eyes see as we begin to make sense of the new-born reflexes that control much of our muscle motor coordination.

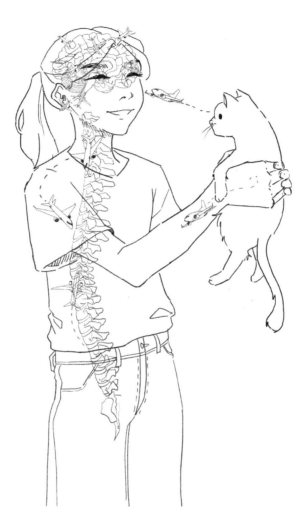

When we receive information from our visual sense, it sets those airplane neural connection patterns in motion. One plane might be carrying information about the incoming information of a cat's size and color. The brain then processes that and sends information to our muscles for how much force to use to lift the cat based on our perceptions of the size. Next, our proprioceptors and skin stretch receptors send information back to the brain to let us know if we need to adjust our calculations. We even calculate our feedback from our postural muscles to know if we are counterbalancing appropriately as we increase the lever of our arms to lift the cat and move our center of gravity. When our eye muscles don't develop correctly, we may have double vision, or the cat may appear to vibrate, making it difficult to perceive. We may not know how far away the cat is so that we can posturally stabilize ourselves efficiently. If we are highly visually distracted by an over-responsive visual scanning system influenced by trauma, we may not notice if the cat moves from friendly and compliant to bored and ready to scratch us.

As we look at the neuroscience of development, the eyes bring information into the brainstem. Eyes have a large impact on our foundational brain hierarchy. When a person loses brain function, the pupils become fixed and dilated as a sign of loss of brainstem functioning.

As we look at behavior analysis, we see how the ability to see or scan a room helps our nervous system feel safe.

While the eyes do provide a lot of warning sensory input, the other senses will often heighten when the eyes are impacted early. For example, studies have shown that the senses of hearing and smell appear amplified when a person is blind. And when the eyes are not stimulated early in development, as can be the case with trauma, the person can become cortically blind, meaning they perceive light but cannot interpret visual images.

When I check for eye movement, I assess if the eyes can move in a smooth pursuit. Can they look up without neck movement? Does the child run around the room upon entry or have difficulty copying from the front classroom screen? How is their reading, eye contact, and finding objects in a drawer or messy room? Are they easily distracted during fine motor tasks? A simple "follow my finger" test to assess if the child can look up, down, left, and right without using neck muscles will indicate visual muscle health.

Suggestions for therapeutic activities that help with **muscular movement of the eyes** taken from the KALMAR app:

- **Modify the environment** to provide external support for visual input. Examples would be corrective lenses or positioning visual tasks in a more focal location. Decrease visual clutter and ask the individual if they prefer different colors or have preferences for warm or cool lights.

- **Position the individual on their back** (to keep the head still) and use a laser light or flashlight to visually track on the ceiling. Practice moving eyes left to right, side to side, up to down, and in circular movements to strengthen the eye muscles.

- **Turn off lights and shine a flashlight** (spotlight) on the desired area of attention to highlight the area and block out the distracting peripheral visual input.

- **Utilize different seating positions** that require looking up for brief periods of time, such as on their belly, under a desk, or over a ball or bolster. This will strengthen the neck muscles, which will impact the eye muscles reflexively.

- **Wearing a hoodie or ball cap** to decrease peripheral vision. Focal vision tends to be more calming, whereas items attended to in our periphery tend to be more alerting.

CHAPTER 4

The Diencephalon and Cerebellum

The diencephalon and cerebellum are parts of the brain that control arousal, physiological homeostasis, rhythm, and coordination. These important centers mediate our sleep/wake rhythms and how much activation our body exhibits. The diencephalon mediates attention to tasks such as fine motor and gross motor activities. The cerebellum helps mediate the smoothness of these activities. It helps us match motor plans and execute them with automaticity. The cerebellum is incredibly complex and dense. Nearly half of our neurons are located in this region, and they have connections to many other parts of the brain and body. However, these neurons are more specialized than neurons in other areas of the brain. They are also formed very early in development. Because of this, there tends to be less plasticity in this region to make quick and easy neural change. While I don't mean this doomily, it helps to have the perspective that change here will be very gradual and require intentionality. From a rehab perspective, it is useful to think of ways we can provide external support for the skills that are mediated in this brain region.

When someone has a diagnosis in the brain that is more visible in nature, such as a cerebellar stroke, we understand that we need to provide stretching exercises to keep them able to move, and we provide structural braces to help them be in a position to optimally interact with their environment. We provide wheelchairs and communication software to assist them with interacting with the world. We lower our body stance to better make eye contact and connect with them. When dealing with a child who presents with regulation, coordination, and rhythmic difficulties, it is helpful to imagine having to brace them and move to be down on their level a bit more in order to successfully rehabilitate them. For diencephalon- and cerebellum-mediated behaviors, rehabilitation may look more like progress than cure. It is important to mindfully match expectations for this brain region.

Functions that are mediated in the diencephalon/cerebellum that occupational therapists can influence include:

- sleep
- gross motor skills
- fine motor skills
- engagement (withdrawal/lethargic or overly active/constantly moving)
- sensory integrative processing.

Sleep

When I assess difficulty with sleep, I ask if they have difficulty falling asleep or staying asleep. If they have trouble falling asleep, they may need sensory or relational support. If they wake up in the middle of the night, I am curious about whether there is a physical imbalance causing a need to urinate frequently, or a side effect of medications either wearing off or causing nightmares. I wonder if it is the same time each night and if that maybe coincides with something startling in the environment. Would changing the lighting, fragrances, bed position, or sleep textiles make a difference?

Are they afraid of the dark or do they seem fearful of bedtime? Would a night light or walkie-talkie to know a caregiver is immediately accessible be helpful? Are they often tired during the day or fall asleep unexpectedly? Is the rest they are getting even restful? Do they need to have a sleep study to determine if they have sleep apnea (a disruption of the breathing pattern when sleeping)?

Sleep is where we refresh and renew. Our bodies restore and replenish during sleep. When we have a physical injury or emotional stress, our bodies are designed to desire more sleep so that we can heal. Something I found interesting is childhood "growing pains." While my own children were in this phase of development, a friend of mine reminded me that the bones grow first and stretch out the muscles and tendons. So, as the body is literally growing, those muscles and tendons are being stretched. That gave me a bit more empathy towards my own son's "growing pains." But I was still frustrated that they seemed only to happen at night. It felt like he was manipulating the situation to not have to go to bed. Then I remembered that the body grows...at night. This realization helped me reframe his behavior as an unmet need and physical pain rather than a manipulative tactic to not sleep. This reframe then made me reconsider how my clients sleep. Children *need* sleep. So why do so many of them not want to sleep? Why do some kids fall asleep immediately while others can take much longer and even sleep very little in extreme cases? Almost every time, it comes back to physical sensations and felt-safety.

When we view sleep through the lens of trauma, we further realize that much of childhood trauma takes place at night, when a child is defenseless. Closing their eyes is letting down their defenses. Having patience and compassion can help the child feel as if their concerns are validated and the adult is willing to listen and help protect them. Just because an adult *says* it is safe does not mean that it feels safe to the child. Memories and strong association patterns do not change overnight. It can take months and even years for a child who was abused at night to feel safe in their new environment.

When a child experiences violence and chaos in their developmental years, their bodies may adapt to "feel" safe in that chaos. I've heard examples of children who need to create chaos before bed by throwing bedroom items into piles so that it is visually familiar to their early childhood. They would rather sleep on a pile of clothes than in their designer-sheet-covered bed. If there was a lot of verbal or physical abuse in their past, they may instigate arguments to match the early pattern of intense emotional or physical activation before the release that follows where they physically collapse. For my clients who present this way, I am curious with the caregiver if we can allow them to have a messy room or if we can engage in some playful roughhousing before bedtime to ease them into this transition from awake to sleep.

For most children, a soothing bedtime routine is sufficient to help them calm to sleep. For others, we need to rethink what is familiar to them and what *feels* safe to them. Then we work in the context of a connected caregiver relationship to slowly introduce new ways to calm down and allow our bodies to rest. For some children, nap times are a good time to practice this skill. Trying different sleeping positions, textures, stories, and routines each day before the child is exhausted can be helpful when looking for ways to adjust previous routines and patterns.

It is important to consider caregiver capacity when children do not sleep regularly or soundly. As any caregiver of a newborn can confirm, when the child doesn't sleep well, the caregiver doesn't sleep well. When both individuals are exhausted, it can be difficult to communicate verbally as both may move down the arousal continuum a bit when the base arousal is exhaustion. Normalizing non-traditional sleep patterns and habits for both the child and the caregiver is beneficial when there has been early trauma or adversity.

Suggestions for therapeutic activities that help with **sleep** taken from the KALMAR app:

- **Allowing a pet to share the bed** or even floor can provide an element of comfort and perceived protection. Pets can also provide soft fur and a steady heartbeat to co-regulate at bedtime.

- **Special sleep music**, white noise, or noise-canceling headphones can help an individual who is easily distracted by background noises. A familiar sound can bring an element of predictability that can calm the brainstem from attending to every new novel input.

- **Modified lighting** can help with melatonin levels. Use a timer adaptation device that allows a light to remain on for a certain duration, such as 30 minutes, and then automatically turns off once the timer is up and the child is asleep. These can commonly be found around holiday light decorations. Graduated sunrise lights are good for gradual sleep and wake cycles.

- **Allowing the child to sleep with another being** such as a sibling, pet, or caregiver when appropriate can be helpful for the child who is afraid of being alone. A mattress on the floor of the caregiver's room can provide appropriate boundaries while maintaining proximity for felt-safety and connection.

- **Leaving doors open** or providing a tent or closed environment when the room cannot be private can ease the fears of a child who doesn't want to be left alone.

Gross motor skills

As we further consider skills influenced by the diencephalon and cerebellum, we look at gross motor skills and the ability to coordinate a thought or intent into a movement pattern. Developmentally, we mature from our spinal cord towards our fingertips and toes. We must first have core stability to have the refined movements of being able to engage our arms and eventually complete dexterous tasks with our hands. Gross motor skills are complex in the number of processes involved. When we do an activity analysis of gross motor skills, we discover that our vestibular sense must engage to tell structures in our diencephalon where our head is in relation to gravity. With this knowledge, our postural muscles will then engage and provide the stability and support needed to counterbalance the movements that are about to challenge the vestibular system of our body. For example, tilt your head back while standing and notice how your stomach muscles engage to keep you from falling back and how your arms might want to lift up a bit to act as a counterweight to help you balance. Now tilt your head forward and notice how your backside engages to prevent you from falling forward.

Once you have stabilized your body, the brain must tell the muscles a sequence of engaging and relaxing. If your quads and hamstrings engaged at the same time, you would simply be immobile with muscle cramps. It's the timing and rhythm of the sequence of relaxing and engaging that propels the leg forward in a gross motor movement pattern such as walking. If this rhythm is off, if the cerebellum does not coordinate this rhythm, it is difficult to progress forward.

As occupational therapists, we look for patterns in that neural processing. Using the lens of sequential development, we then trace the patterns back sequentially to find the part that is not functioning optimally, with hopes of rehabilitation. It is with this multisystem complexity lens that we look at gross motor skills. If we do not have good vestibular integration for balance, it won't matter how strong our muscles are. If our muscles are weak, it won't matter how great our balance is. So how do we know where to start? We can look at this two ways. One is by asking ourselves what we can easily adapt. If we brace or support the muscles easily, we can try that and see if something simple can make a difference. Maybe we give them support while we do the home exercise program that will build up the muscle strength over time.

Maybe we look at it completely differently and see that the child has poor nutrition and therefore is unable to engage in gross motor tasks because of lack of the protein building blocks or calcium that provide the cellular stability to fire the muscles.

When we think back to the diencephalon's influence on arousal levels and attention, we also want to consider if the person is able to sustain focus or interest in the activity long enough to learn or complete it.

From a physical rehab perspective, practice and repeated movements are one of the best ways to improve gross motor skills once we have established the building blocks that are required for this skill. While engaged in these repetitive practice movements, there are some things we can do therapeutically that will improve the rehab outcome.

We can make the gross motor skill easier by making it even bigger. If you try to catch a large ball, it is easier to see in your visual field. It requires less distance and precision of arm movement to catch a large ball compared to a smaller ball. This means that there is less chance for error, and thus the client receives more positive feedback to influence motivation to continue the therapeutic exercise of tossing and catching a ball. A soft or mildly deflated ball will move through the air more slowly and is less likely to bounce out of the client's arms upon catching. Sport balls with tactile interest provide more sensory input for the tactile system. This provides information to the tactile receptive neurons to *feel* the catching a ball.

As I consider other modifications I could make, I think about including other sensory receptors. Could adding lights to the ball help? Could they sustain visual attention to the ball longer if it has a flashing light inside? What if I added a jingle bell inside so the client could hear where it was coming from? How heavy is the ball? A heavy ball will provide more proprioceptive input, which is the sensation that tells you where you are in relation to other objects. Or would a lighter ball be better because the client has muscle weakness and is unable to maintain the muscle strength for a heavier ball?

What if our gross motor skill is riding a bike? How do I think through how to modify that activity? I again begin with activity analysis. What is involved with riding a bike? I need rhythm (brainstem). I need good balance (cerebellum). I need coordination (cerebral cortex). I need visual skills (ocular motor cortex). I need proprioceptive receptors and nerves that give direction and feedback on how my limbs are moving. I need muscle strength (muscles). I need to know what direction to go and how to navigate traffic (executive function). With so many areas involved, I once again ask myself, is there some way I can scaffold or build support from the outside that will be helpful? Can I provide an adaptive bicycle that helps decrease the need for balance or motor control? Can I provide a buddy, so they don't have to navigate the traffic and directions?

Once I have considered ways to provide external help, I then look at the individual skills and consider them through the lens of sequential brain development. Since rhythm is in the brainstem, I probably need to work on that first. I can do this by playing with drums, nursery rhymes, pop and rap music (if they are older), and simple hand connection games like pat-a-cake. As I choose the activity, I'm also looking through the lens of age appropriateness. I can't play pat-a-cake with a ten-year-old. But I can ask them to teach pat-a-cake to a two-year-old. I can create a special handshake between the two of us that is practiced often. I can play drums on pots and pans or even a table. Once I have good rhythm and timing, I will begin to move forward in brain development to work on balance and coordination. I might have the child practice simply standing on one foot, hopping from side to side to get some rhythm and coordination engaged along with the balance. I might have them practice a bicycle move while they are on their back so that they can be working on rhythm and coordination without the complexity of balance since most of their weight is supported by the floor as they begin to practice this movement.

If a child experiences neglect early in life when the body is developing and ready to learn skills such as riding a bike, they may not have had the opportunities to experience and learn these skills. When a child is confined to small spaces, they do not have the opportunities to stretch their muscles and limbs and practice these gross motor patterns. Our bones become stronger as we put weight on them and create small, healthy micro-fractures. Without this weight-bearing movement, people who experience early neglect can even have soft bones or lack stability once they begin to move about.

If a child grows up in a chaotic environment, they may have relied heavily on being able to move quickly to get out of harm's way. These children get excess practice in some of these gross motor movement patterns and overly rely on them for felt protection and navigation of their environment. Some people overly rely on their gross motor movements and are in constant motion. They have difficulty sitting still and allowing the body to calm for more cognitive processing. For some, they need to add proprioceptive input to calm the gross motor movement reliance.

For the KALMAR app, I refer to gross motor concerns as falling often, poor balance, difficulty crossing the midline, toe walking, W-sitting, difficulty with sports techniques, and holding breath during activity.

Frequent falling could be caused by weak core musculature or difficulty with balance. We can strengthen muscles through the home program, but if the balance is off, those muscles won't know how to engage and relax in the rhythm that creates the movement patterns that are desired. So we would begin with balance. Maybe it is as simple as engaging the vestibular receptors through small rhythmic repetitive exercises such as a rocker board or swinging on a swing while the postural muscles engage and relax to keep our head steady. Maybe we do dancing and bring music into the therapy session because music and balance work well together. It's difficult to dance or bee bop along to music without good balance. Even the nerve that innervates balance is called the vestibulocochlear nerve, meaning balance and hearing are inherently tied together.

If a child doesn't cross the midline, they will be unable to complete many gross motor skills. Most gross motor skills involve both sides of the body and movement across the sagittal plane. Throwing and catching a ball often requires twisting at the torso. Dancing and simply reaching for a glass on a shelf can require the left arm to move towards the right shoulder. Keeping in mind how much is involved in the seemingly simplest movements, we can see how visual fields will change and muscles will coordinate flexing and extending in smooth patterns, as the different sides of the brain that mediate these muscles on the opposite sides of the body engage. When a client can't cross their midline fluidly, it can cause difficulty with simple daily-life activities. Many movements that involve balance also require coordinated movement across the transverse plane. For example, the left arm and right leg bend while the right arm and left leg extend in order to walk or run in a forward pattern. As we look at how balance and coordination are foundational to our daily activities, it is easier to understand how these activities can be more difficult and even impossible when we have difficulty with the cerebellum. If a child is unable to have good balance in a chair, they will have even more trouble with desk work such as handwriting or even holding a book steady to read. If their eyes do not easily cross the midline, they will have difficulty with reading text across the page. This is yet another example of how we cannot do higher-level tasks without the base brain level functioning optimally.

One of my favorite ways to practice building new neural connections for crossing the midline is to sit on the ground with legs crossed in a pretzel manner while the child uses a writing tool to make a large rainbow that stretches from one side of the body to the other where it appears that the child is sitting under the rainbow. Standing very close to a wall or marker board and making rainbows, figure eights, and circles is another great way to practice crossing the midline. As I explore the various new school movement programs, many of the movements remind me of Tai Chi, which is another excellent and engaging way to encourage my clients to practice crossing their midlines.

When a child engages in a lot of toe walking and W-sitting, I become curious about their muscle tone. Often, kids who walk on their toes a lot are looking for increased proprioceptive input to know where their foot is in relation to the floor. Sometimes it is because their calf muscles are too tight, or they have poor postural control or balance. A simple experiment I have caregivers practice is to stand up on your toes and take a step. Notice how your body moves forward almost without effort. If you have ever worn high heels, you may have noticed how difficult it can be to stop once you begin moving forward. This is because being on your toes shifts your center of gravity and propels your body forward, compensating for weak core muscles and using less effort to get you started moving forward. When we W-sit, we widen our base of support so that our core does not have to engage as strongly. This widened base of support also helps us be more stable, like the legs of a tripod expanding to hold up a heavy camera. Holding our breath is another way to stabilize our core. When we hold our breath, our core muscles engage. They remain contracted until the out-breath.

Most sport activities involve coordinated gross motor skills. Asking how my clients perform in sports can give me information on their gross motor abilities as well as their social abilities. This question can also assist me in knowing what community activities the caregivers have attempted as well as the child's possible interests, strengths, and talents. If they struggled in football, lacrosse, and basketball but did well in swimming and cross-country, I wonder if individual sports are more comfortable for them. Is tennis preferred to baseball because they do best with consistent exertion instead of the sudden spurts? Or is baseball better because it can be more predictable? These are the types of patterns I'm trying to find for my clients. I often ask my ponderings out loud and see if there is any revelation for the caregiver. So often I become curious, and the caregiver is the one that sees the pattern before I do. It is sometimes easier for them to find these patterns as they walk through their week once I've planted the seed of curiosity for them.

Suggestions for therapeutic activities that help with **gross motor skills** taken from the KALMAR app:

- **Drumming** helps with motor planning due to the strong auditory, proprioceptive, predictive, and rhythmic nature.

- Have clients engage in large motor, **heavy farm chores** such as cleaning stalls, hauling water, and grooming large animals. Exercise with proprioceptive emphasis (crash and bump) helps provide additional input when practicing motor plans.

- **Recreational outlets** that involve proprioception and repetitive movements such as swimming and basketball provide a lot of engaging and rewarding repetition, needed for new motor plans.

- **Sensory-rich exploration** and mindfulness such as walking, hiking, and biking can help with gross motor skills by calming the brainstem through the repetitive nature. Yet they often provide small doses of change to help with carry-over to other tasks.

- **Planned and sequenced movements** such yoga/pilates, core strengthening, and balance beams provide good predictive structure to improve gross motor skills.

Fine motor skills

Fine motor skills add refinement to the gross motor skills. Fine motor skills are built upon the stability of the core. They require balance and postural support to independently move the outermost extremities. Proximal stability allows for distal mobility. If we do not have a good base of support, we will not be able to execute refined fine motor skills.

For the KALMAR app, I refer to fine motor skills as the ability to cut, color, put keys in a lock, use utensils, play instruments, and use hand muscles.

In her podcast SpIRiTed Conversations with pediatric occupational therapists Cory Dundon and Michelle Maunder, Tracy Stackhouse once mentioned how humans are made to create. She explained how we have an internal desire to interact with our environment. When we see a hill, we want to climb it. When we see a ball, we want to throw or kick it. When we see small objects, we want to manipulate them; indeed, some of us need to fidget with something even when we are presented with the task of sitting still. We use our fingers, and especially our unique opposing thumbs, to create beautiful works of art, enhance the flavors and textures of our food, and create functional and aesthetically pleasing places to dwell. We use our hands to work the land, to hold the tools those hands previously created, and maneuver vehicles that take us to places of exploration. We use our fine motor skills to communicate in written form and access items that give us independence. We often use our hands in rhythmic, repetitive, brainstem-calming ways such as doodling, picking, knitting, drumming, or flapping. We use our fingers to touch those who are in relationship with us. When we do not have good fine motor skills, we miss out on opportunities for self-soothing, self-expression, and the richness of being human.

Fine motor skills rely heavily on the rhythm and coordination of the muscles and the timing and thoughts for recalculation. When there is a misfire in the timing of the muscle activation and relaxation, we see difficulty in the form of shaky movements, over- and under-targeting of interacting with objects, and inability to grasp and release in smooth rhythm. This makes the act of engaging in fine motor skills more difficult. To help with this, we can increase the information that the brain receives through intensity and work to externally brace the task. We can add glue, or a product called Wikki Stix to the outsides of a coloring page to provide an elevated boundary to keep the color within the lines. We can offer adaptive scissors that are spring-loaded to assist with the motor planning of a cutting task. We can allow more time to complete a task. We can decrease the number expected for task completion, such as only writing out five math problems and allowing the other 15 to be solved verbally, to build endurance while fostering confidence. We can use our own bodies to provide rhythm through our breath, through our own finger, hand, and leg movements that can be mimicked by the client. Examples would be rhythmically passing a ball, receiving this co-rhythm through riding a horse, or adding other sensation support such as lights or sound to help guide the client through an activity. We can encourage the client to sit on a swing or rocking chair that is under our rhythmic influence while they complete a fine motor task.

When we view fine motor skills through the lens of adversity, we find that people who live in adversity often lack experience, modeling, and relational teaching of how to use their hands skillfully. Much of fine motor rehabilitation is providing the opportunity to practice while scaffolding for success. Tasks that provide proprioceptive input can also increase the information being gathered to intensify the learning. Adding proprioceptive weight or resistance can slow the process down to allow the brain further time for integration. An example of this is writing on sandpaper instead of a dry erase board or using crayons and pencils instead of smooth ballpoint pens and markers. I've used fettuccine and rolled putty to teach cutting skills because that is another easy way to increase the resistance and proprioceptive input. Once the client has learned the motor planning sequence with the increased proprioceptive feedback, it becomes a matter of repeated practice and repetition to build the neural motor memory.

Fine motor skills are a form of expression. They are a way we can control our surroundings. When we struggle with proficiency in fine motor skills, we may be easily frustrated by a lack of control or ability to creatively express ourselves. It's difficult to play an instrument, paint a picture, or knit a scarf without skilled use of our hands. This frustration of perceived failure can lead to rejection or refusal to attempt fine motor activities. Recognizing this, it is important for the therapist to find ways to make fine motor practice engaging, interesting, and meaningful from the client's perspective. I once saw a Far Side cartoon that depicted an aerobics class in Hell. The caption was "Three more, two more, one more, okay!... Five million leg lifts right leg first!... Ready, set!...". That cartoon is often visualized in my brain as I engage in therapeutic exercise. I never want to be that guy. I don't want to spend my life counting. I want to spend my life *doing*. I want to engage my clients in purposeful activity. Sure, I could lift my leg a million times. It will certainly make me stronger. But if I can engage a peer or sibling to kick that ball into a net repeatedly with me, I've added a really fun relational aspect that lights up a little more of the brain in my imaginary fMRI fireworks show.

Suggestions for therapeutic activities that help with **fine motor skills** taken from the KALMAR app:

- Consider **modifications** specific to fine motor skills such as adaptive writing utensils, spring-loaded scissors, or building up handles to help with grasp.

- **Decrease the workload** so that the individual has a sense of completion and success instead of overwhelm.

- Fine motor **dexterity and strength exercises** can build muscle strength, control, and success of motor planning movements. Putty, slime, dough, and soft water toys can be very motivating ways to encourage hand strength.

- A **weighted wrist cuff** can provide increased proprioceptive feedback and decrease tremors that make fine motor tasks difficult.

- Make activities **purposeful** and clear to help the individual have buy-in to the functional outcome goal.

Engagement (withdrawal/lethargic or overly active/constantly moving)

Our lives are meant to ebb and flow and not remain in a stagnant state of arousal. We need to be able to match our mental and physical states dependent upon our ever-changing environment. To do this, our nervous system is constantly monitoring internal and external cues for a sense of felt-safety and chemically coding that information through our neural networks based on that felt-safety assessment. This sense of felt-safety is influenced both by our current experience and our memories of past experiences. Because of this, we must factor in past traumatic experiences as we assess a client's ability to appropriately engage in daily activities. My clients who present with blank stares, withdrawal, robotic compliance, lack of response to pain, or frequent undiagnosed ailments like headaches and fatigue fall into Dr. Perry's dissociative arousal continuum briefly referenced at the beginning of this book. Clients who present with overactivity, excessive talking, difficulty settling down, and frequent aggression fall into the hyper-arousal side of the continuum. A point of clarification I find helpful is to realize that the continuum is not a pendulum with two opposite sides. Both dissociation and hyperarousal are nervous system states that are coded neurologically as feeling unsafe. This results in neurochemistry that facilitates the body to go into a protective mode.

When we subconsciously interpret these codes as if fighting is our best chance of survival, we exhibit our protective responses in more aggressive, outward patterns. However, when we interpret these codes as fleeing being our best chance of survival, we exhibit our protective responses in more dissociative, inward patterns. Thus, both the hyper-arousal and dissociative continuums are responses that escalate as our sense of felt-safety decreases.

When I have a client that is working on goals in this area, it is usually because they are stuck in a high arousal state (which could look like either fight *or* freeze) or they have difficulty with the rhythm of moving between the states. Often, they move through these states too quickly. This is conveyed as "they go from zero to 60 without warning" or "they are like a light switch—either on or off." Often my goal for engagement is written as "self-regulation" or "ability to match their action activation with the social context of the environment." Clients I work with often don't have the practice of smoothly moving between activation levels because they didn't have a responsive and attuned caregiver to guide them in their toddler years. They didn't have safe social environments to practice social interactions alongside a lovingly instructive caregiver. So we must go back developmentally and help them practice co-regulation before self-regulation.

For this goal, it is important to view the arousal level through the lens of both environmental and emotional background in addition to current context. If we desire for the client to be able to "read the room" and adjust to the social context, we must first be able to "read their background" and understand what other background context they are dealing with. Being trauma aware and having a relationship with the client where I can know what happened before our session can be helpful. I once heard of a child who is in the foster system and has few possessions being told, "I'm going to wait for you in the car while you have this fit. If you don't leave the playground now with your siblings, I'll just leave all your things to be donated for another little girl to enjoy." This type of harsh punishment makes me cringe for any child. This child's past experiences with loss, abandonment, and feeling that her worth may be tied to material items makes this even more horrifying. So, for this client, I offer that metaphor of the brace for a child diagnosed with cerebral palsy. This child needs outside support. My treatment is to educate this caregiver on the background of how this child may perceive this situation very differently than the adult. While the adult may be thinking of getting home to get dinner on the table and keep everyone on a schedule, the child was being developmentally appropriate with not wanting to leave a fun activity. The proprioceptive and vestibular input of the playground may have felt therapeutic to them and they weren't ready to leave it. When your sense of timing, rhythm, and sensory input is impaired, transitions are very difficult. With the added history of loss, it was incredibly difficult for this child to follow the simple request of leaving the playground and getting into the car.

For this client, I instruct the parent on the importance of known expectations, transitional support, extra time, and flexibility on the part of the caregiver. The cerebellum influences timing and coordination, so when a child has advanced warning of a sequence of events via a visual calendar, an auditory rhythm/rhyme of sequence, or calmly and respectfully articulated clock countdowns, it helps prepare the cerebellum to respond when the moment arrives. Having transitional support could look like the caregiver assisting with gathering the play items. Simply holding the bag open or mirroring the child as they grab the shovels and you grab the pails can be helpful. When extensive practice is needed to form those pathways of leaving a preferred event, having a co-regulator and someone to parallel with you is necessary. Allowing extra time gives both the caregiver and the child space to make mistakes and re-calibrate the coordination of the motor planning events needed to gather personal belongings. Without these supports, the child may not be independently successful at gathering the supplies and heading to the car. When they fail this task and are then punished with a threat that triggers past hurts, things can escalate quickly for both the caregiver and the child.

One of the ways I help clients in my therapy room with engagement is through playful practice. I ask the caregiver to cue up a Spotify playlist with 120–140 bpm instrumental music. Then I cue up 60–80 bpm music on my own phone. I add the word "instrumental" to help monitor inappropriate content for a pediatric client population. I have created a therapeutic playlist called "Marti's Therapy Songs" that can be found on Spotify. Here, I have a few fast songs and a few slow songs that I use in my therapy spaces.

Our motor planning is like a pendulum. Our first walking steps are exaggerated and overshot to the right side, left side, front, back, and even top to bottom. It is through repetition and mirrored learning that we begin to walk in a straight, coordinated line. We don't learn to walk by being told how to walk or simply watching others walk. Our engagement is the same. We first move between really calm and really activated. Because of this, therapy must also be a wide pendulum of experience. In the beginning, I will play more fast music than slow music. Most of my clients are much more practiced and comfortable in the fast zones, and I first need to match their energy to help establish a relational connection. While the music is playing fast, I provide outside manipulation of the movement of their body. I find a bolster swing or a Lycra hammock to be the easiest way for me to accomplish this. A therapy ball is another option. However, sometimes the children I work with get too silly on the ball and flop around unsafely or they simply bounce right off. The bolster swing gives the extra therapeutic bonus of strengthening core postural muscles while in a posture that is easier to achieve for most kids. The Lycra hammock is even more contained as it snuggles around them and thus encourages less child-initiated movement so they "feel" my rhythm even more.

Once the child is physically supported upon the vestibular equipment, I move their body in rhythm with the music. In the beginning, I bring structure with slow music. But only for a few quick, 3–6-second bursts. I'll ask the caregiver to have a fast song cued up on their phones next to us. I do this intentionally so that the child is connecting in a positive, even eager, way with the caregiver. I may leave this music on for 5–10 seconds since it is where most children are most comfortable at first. Then I will say "SLOW!" and the caregiver pauses the music on their phone while my slow Mozart music begins to play on my phone. I am playful at first and use my posture, tone of voice, and my own rhythm next to the vestibular equipment to bring the child down *with* me. I don't leave them here long if it isn't a natural state for them. Within 3–6 seconds, I will excitedly announce, "FAST" and the focus is then directed to the caregiver for some gleeful fast bouncing on the equipment to the tempo of the faster music.

After I introduce this concept of feeling fast and slow rhythms, I can expand the time between the sensations. When the child starts to integrate my rhythm and timing, I give them control of the fast/slow timing announcement. This gives me an opportunity to therapeutically observe the child's felt-sense of timing. I become curious and make mental notes of how quickly they switch. I notice how long they stay in one state compared to another. I begin to ease my external input and assess if they are able to keep the beat in other parts of their body such as their hands or their neck. This is a wonderfully therapeutic activity that not only engages the child to allow the therapist a glimpse of their internal rhythm, but also allows a playful engagement to practice the movement between high and low activation while maintaining relationship and pleasant engagement.

Another great way to practice this up-and-down rhythmic interaction is with drums. In my clinic, I have several types of drums. I find that the children who tend to be anxious or high-energy gravitate towards the higher-pitched drums. These drums tend to match their internal state a bit more and help them keep in a higher alert zone while being able to be playful with rhythmic beats. This is an activity that factors in several therapeutic inputs. The high pitch of the drum has an alerting quality. However, if we do a slow percussion rhythm, that is a calming input. I use this analysis therapeutically when I am looking for activities that will be respectful to the client and resonate with them in their current level of functioning, while, in tandem, inviting them to join my co-regulation of adjusting their internal activation to be manipulated to better fit my interpretation of the social construct. When I don't attempt to find a way to match the client, I have more difficulty with motivational buy-in to my therapeutic attempts. I've tried simply introducing a deep-sounding bass drum to a highly anxious child and it sometimes appears to make them even more anxious. However, if I myself am banging on the deeper drum while they bang the higher drum, I can adjust my own actions to better make them feel mirrored. This can be described as empowering and regulating them as I move towards connecting and relating to them. I first give them the drum to "go wild." After a brief introduction of focused attention so that they feel "seen," I then begin to follow their lead with my own drum. Since I have the bass, our bodies tend to lean into that sound more than the higher pitches. Once I gain that initial connection, I can begin to influence our little personal drum circle and get playful with how I increase or decrease the tempo. Once engaged, I can begin to play with slowly moving up and down activation levels. This allows me to be observant and watch for clues as the child begins to get out of their comfort zone. They may become disengaged, ignore me, leave the drum, or become aggressive with their playing. When I can, I mirror them and see if they come back in sync with me. Or maybe I can feel something in my own body that leads me to "feel" what is going on for them. For particularly difficult-to-read children, it can be beneficial to record a session and go back and look for clues that you may have missed at the moment. Some children shift their eye gaze away or move their body posture away from you in the moments before they escalate on the arousal continuum.

Another therapeutic tip is to become a rhythm detective in moments of apparent distress. When a child appears "out of control" and is increasing in activity and potentially more aggressive-type movements, I watch for the cerebellar clue of rhythm again. When the cerebellum is activated to provide calm, the movement is rhythmic. It's like a clue to me that the child's network planes are able to land. I simply need to give them ground control clearance. Rhythm tells me that the child is able to access their level of coordination. An "out-of-control" child typically lacks rhythm and coordination. This is a clue to me that they are seeking something that their body isn't currently able to integrate or understand. When I see this, I first think of basic needs. Does the child feel safe? Is there a hidden threat that I can't see? Sometimes the plane is hijacked, and the child doesn't know how to communicate the distress in the moment. That plane that is trying to make smooth, coordinated movements is not running in the correct flight pattern through the cerebellum.

An example of hidden threat is when I worked with a child whose fun-loving uncle would hold him down and tickle him. This child did not find it playful and fun, yet the uncle continued to interact in a way that did not feel good to the child because the child would giggle and squeal out of stress that was perceived as delight. The uncle meant well but failed to see that the giggles were actually signs of alarm for this child. Unaware of this, when I was working in a school setting to decrease the amount of pressure that this child put on to the paper, I felt very clever when I suggested he simply "tickle the paper" instead of pressing so hard. I even gave a nice little example as I placed the thin paper on the palm of his hand and demonstrated the tickle compared with "too hard." This child began screaming non-word sounds and hid under his desk. I could not engage him by talking. I could not get him to even look in my direction. I had zero context for this apparent meltdown. His connected and attuned teacher rushed over and asked for context. Baffled, I replayed the scene as I experienced it. She was able to put the scenario into the context of his uncle and assured the child that not only do we not have to tickle the paper, but also paper does not have feelings and would not be hurt by our crayons. Although I didn't know *why* he was distressed, his lack of rhythm led me to find his connected caregiver to help him co-regulate back to safety.

Sometimes I have no context because the child isn't able to verbalize it with me. In these situations, I try to determine if the child's basic internal physical needs are met. Are they tired? Are they hungry? Do they need to have a bowel movement? When I can't identify an internal stress response, I get curious about the sensory environment. Is something too loud for them? Is there an unpleasant scent or a too bright light? What is the temperature? Is there a person nearby that they seem to be fearful of? It doesn't matter if I assess the room and find it safe and sensory pleasing to *my* nervous system. I need it to feel safe and sensory pleasing to the *child's* nervous system. If I'm going to work in the cerebellum, that means I bring my own rhythm to the therapeutic moment. Maybe I hum softly or tap my legs to a soft rhythmic beat. I'm careful not to block the child's perceived exit from the room (even though I may have a plan to intercept them at the door if needed). I might sit next to them and rock back and forth or bring in an animal like a therapy dog or rabbit and rhythmically pet the animal myself before inviting the client to join me. I might try something unexpected and toss a soft pillow or ball playfully in their direction. Sometimes this is enough to distract their attention to the present moment and engage them in some reciprocal play with me. A balloon is an excellent choice for back-and-forth play because it moves slower and requires less coordination for accuracy. When the cerebellum is not in optimal function, requiring less coordination can be better. If this is still too much, a Slinky, blown bubbles, handheld objects that can slowly fade between colors, or other slow-moving rhythmic items provide a nice interaction that begins to stimulate and integrate the cerebellum so that the child can better monitor their arousal activation level.

Changing locations and full-body movement can also be a very helpful way to influence our arousal and engagement. Marching down the hallway, walking or running dependent upon energy level, or a quick dance break can be a nice way to meet a child in an activated state and then bring them back to the needed state within a mirrored movement relationship.

For some children, simply hearing our voice can be too complicated when they are trying to coordinate their activity level to the social milieu. With older children, I've found texting to be a nice compromise that decreases the need to process so much non-verbal body language and tone. Of course, text is not ideal for regular communication as a lot can be misunderstood without these other cues. But simple requests such as "Please put your shoes in the closet" or "Please help me chop some veggies for dinner" can seem much less threatening when texted for a child who is disconnected. It also gives them a little more time to formulate the motor plan to accomplish the requested task. It's a strategy that can't hurt and it might help.

The powerful formula for self-regulation is to first make sure their biological and emotional needs are met while matching their energy and bringing their rhythm up or down in the context of relationship. I'm optimistic for systemic change, with the next parenting generation having the benefit of neuroscience and great leaders and educators like my fellow TBRI practitioners, Brené Brown, Robyn Gobbel, Tracy Stackhouse, Dr. Perry, and so many other therapists I work with, teaching the science of more attuned ways of parenting.

Suggestions for therapeutic activities that help with **engagement (withdrawal/lethargy or overly active/constantly moving)** taken from the KALMAR app:

- **Bubbles** are a great therapeutic activity for ages nine months to 109 years. The whimsical and unexpected yet slow and rhythmic path of the bubbles make it a just-right alert/calm activity to share with clients.

- **Drumming and rhythmic music** can be a way to connect a group or couple in a matched rhythm and co-regulatory activity.

- Try to find an **animal that matches the energy tempo** of the client. Ask the client which animal they "relate to" and pair them with that animal if possible. Chickens can match a very energetic client while a rabbit or goat will be calmer. A snake can be great for a highly alert but dissociative adolescent. It moves slowly but provides that alertness of, well, being a snake.

- Give a **sense of control** as much as possible and provide a calming space when needed. If possible, construct the calming environment in such a way that two people could sit side by side to co-regulate. When an individual experiences trauma, it is often in the context of a controlling relationship. Allowing the individual control over the proximity of a co-regulatory activity can help increase their felt-safety.

- **Social Stories™** (Gray, 2000) can be helpful when an individual did not have typical examples of social interactions as a child. They may want to engage with others but lack the understanding and experience of how to engage. A Social Story helps guide them and gives them a script to follow and practice before social interactions are better integrated for the individual.

- **Weaving preferred activities into a non-preferred activity** helps to build a tolerance for the non-preferred activity while providing the motivation for continued endurance of the non-preferred activity.

Sensory integrative processing

I love chatting with OT friends who are just as passionate about helping people who have experienced adversity as I am. Amy Herring Lewis, OTR/L, is one of these friends. She wrote a curriculum called "Powerfully You" (www.powerfullyyou.org) that helps therapists teach people how to better understand their body cues and identify strategies that personally help them better understand their internal and external senses. She loves to study and learn from top therapists in our field. She has a lot of great experience, understanding, and awareness of current trends, models, language, and treatment protocols. Amy and I were discussing neurobiology one day and how so many new therapists are hesitant with sensory strategies because they, like my younger self, think there is some sort of magical formula they don't know about yet. My older self realizes that the magic is unique to each individual. There is no "one size fits all" for sensory strategies. Together, Amy and I are trying to better understand the neurobiology of being human in an effort to assist other practitioners to help clients they work with.

As I studied with Amy, we discussed Tracy Stackhouse's teaching and her SpIRiT model. Tracy is part of a camp in Australia called Camp Jabiru. At this camp, several OTs work with children and learn from them while also learning from each other. During one camp session, OTs discussed the confusion with the definitions surrounding "sensory" language. As the OTs conversed, they began to see a need for clarification. They discussed how **sensory processing** typically refers to the mediation of the lower parts of the brain including the brainstem, cerebellum, and the diencephalon, with initial interpretation in the thalamus, hippocampus, and reticular formation. It conveys a more diffuse process of afferent information coming in through the spinal cord and entering the brainstem with a widespread influence on general arousal and regulatory systems. The word "processing" makes me think of a linear process similar to an assembly line. It is the assembling of many parts into one, just as the nerve receptors bring so many types of information into the brainstem. **Sensory integrative processing** refers to the intermingled connections within the higher parts of the brain in the higher limbic and cortical areas. "Integration" refers to the mechanisms of this loop working together in a beautiful symphony of harmonic sensations geared towards keeping our bodies safe while we engage in purposeful activity. Integration is how we know we are safe and are therefore able to put additional meaning to the experience. Sensory processing is seeing an unexpected rubber snake in our path and jumping and screaming in a response to keep our bodies safe. It is the initial assessment and response before we notice this snake isn't moving and maybe isn't even a dangerous color.

Integration in action is noticed when we anticipate and see a snake in a cage. When we feel safe because we know that the snake has been contained in a glass cage, we can begin to notice how it moves so slowly. We can see the intricate patterns and colors on its skin. With the surprise snake, we maybe only noticed the general shape and our senses alerted us to take action immediately without thought. When the threat is removed, we have the capacity to recall different types of snakes we have seen in the past and compare this one against those past snakes of our memories. We may still be fearful of a snake in the wild, but when all the safety information in our brains is integrated, we can make sense of our sensations to know we can pause and reflect to study more attributes of the potentially fearful snake stimulus. We could possibly touch the skin as it is held by the zookeeper. We might notice if the snake has an odor or makes a noise as it moves.

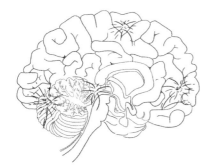

Integrated
Snake Observation

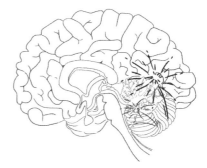

Unexpected
Snake Observation

Sensory integration leads me to think of a networked, air traffic pattern. It is a process of taking information from receptors and seeing how it relates by coordinating and blending senses from a variety of interconnected brain structures. It is the act of experiencing a sensation, formulating an understanding of how that sensation fits into our existing neural framework, and creating a response. A pleasant cup of tea isn't just tasted. The aroma is smelled, the temperature is felt, and we experience it from the cup in our hand all the way down to the liquid in our esophagus. Since we experience our world in dimensional sensation, we create networks that coordinate to become stronger when these paired sensations are repeated. If we have a routine of tea after school with our mom, we may later associate the drinking of tea with pleasant memories of our mom even after we leave her home. For another person, tea may be associated with a time they were abused by someone who drank tea. For them, tea has been integrated and tied to a fear or protective response. Since everyone perceives and interprets their senses uniquely and individually based on their past experiences, it is impossible to give a definitive procedural process to "cure" a diagnosis of sensory integrative processing dysfunction.

Even simple daily routines such as taking a shower can be interpreted uniquely. Some people like to shower during the day, others like to shower at night. In a residential home where showers are scheduled for evenings, the individuals will have different responses based upon their individual sensory preferences that are influenced by their past experiences. They may have even had abuse that happened in a bathroom at night, which would make evening showers even more unsafe feeling for them. As we think through these ideas of preferences, how can we adjust and accommodate within some of our policies and procedures to better consider these individual and unique sensory experiences? Could we offer more choices? Could we simply ask if the person has thoughts, feelings, or ideas around their preferences? Could we view the request of a morning shower as a preference instead of an attempt to manipulate or control? What if the soap in the facility is associated with a previous perpetrator? There are so many new ways to view resistance and non-compliance when we become curious about individual sensory preferences and the past adverse experiences that formed these preferences.

While there is no "magic cure" for sensory-based challenges, there are some commonalities in the way the majority of humans interpret sensations that can be helpful as we look at treatment activities. I call these the "can't hurt, might help" suggestions. I invite the therapist to be curious and try different approaches to gain insight on how a client perceives sensory stimulation and if we can influence their activity level, mood, attention, and understanding of their uniqueness based on how they respond to sensory stimulation.

In my previous book, *The Connected Therapist: Relating Through the Senses* (Smith, 2021), I break down each sense and how it relates to trauma. I've uploaded several handouts to my website (http://www. creativetherapies.com/handouts) that are available for download for more information on what most individuals find calming rather than alerting and how trauma impacts the development of our sensory preferences. We can complete sensory checklists that help us identify patterns of sensory-influenced tendencies. We can use the calm versus alert chart from my previous book to help us plan strategies that influence our client's arousal level while maintaining felt-safety and curiosity. We can then influence recipes of mixing the sensations together for the just-right therapeutic outcome. For example, I use hand-held objects that can light up in sessions when I want a child to be more focused. Understanding that light viewed at midline tends to be more calming, I can use light to adjust the sensory environment for a client who is easily distracted. Just as we put a spotlight on the lead character in the play, we can spotlight the attention of the client. If I am working on a fine motor task with a visually distracted client, I invite them to sit in a Lycra hammock swing while I dim the lights and shine my cell phone flashlight on the task for them. I use color-changing devices to provide a soothing rhythmic flow of color to help a child focus and calm while we are swinging in a slow, rhythmic back-and-forth pattern. I might move the light to a strobe effect (after first confirming they are not a seizure risk). A strobe tends to be more alerting, and I would pair that with upbeat auditory music or a fast, more erratic swinging pattern if I wanted my client to become more energized.

If I know that my client has difficulty with textures, I might introduce challenging textures while on a swing. This pairs the "perceived unsafe" tactile sensation with a preferred sense of felt-safety from the vestibular and proprioceptive input. I might engage the child in singing their favorite song as we play in the shaving cream or slime. Both of these pairings also bring rhythm, repetition, and predictability to the activity. By pairing these sensations, I'm creating new neural associations that touch is not so bad. I'm also watching for cues of overwhelm and giving my client extra time and other offerings of felt-safety. I find that a "safety rag" can be a powerful tool for clients who have difficulty with trust and giving control to an adult. A safety rag is simply a hand towel that is wet on one end and dry on the other. As we play in mud, shaving cream, cookie dough, or paint, I explain to the child that they may access the safety rag at any moment. They may use it every single time the tactile sensation gets on their skin if they wish. Most clients use it generously in the beginning and sparsely by the end of the 50-minute session. Simply having the safety rag allows many of my clients the security and trust to begin to open their window of tolerance a bit.

If I am working to increase a child's tolerance of noises in crowded social environments, I would first provide them with an external support of allowing headphones, ear plugs, or even a hoody sweatshirt. This immediate support signals to the child that I am listening. Their concern is heard and validated. It provides immediate relief to their system while we work together to pair more pleasant interactions that tie overwhelming auditory input within the context of relationship to override the unpleasant heightened arousal level. I can then deconstruct the atmosphere and identify noises I could present in isolation. If the child is over-alerting in the school cafeteria, I can introduce them to half of the sensation before the other children arrive. We can go "behind the scenes" and see/hear the registers beeping and the lunch crew stacking dishes or clanging pots and pans. We can then go out to a recess area with a smaller number of children and listen from a distance to the chatter of excited playmates, without having to simultaneously integrate the other sounds that are specific to the cafeteria. We can then begin lunch before everyone else so that our amount of time in the over-alert environment is limited. Or we put the headphones on the table next to us and put them on and off as needed, with the goal of needing them less each day. We work slowly, with the child's guidance, without shame of going backward or pressure to move forward too quickly. Once the brain has enough experience of repetitions of safety, the client's window of tolerance can open up a bit more until they can enjoy the taste of their food, even when there is a lot of noise in the background.

As I shift from a traditional treatment exercise mode to an observational assessment mode, I might notice that the child is even more agitated on the personal kitchen tour, when the peers are not in attendance. When this is the case, I can get curious about whether the smell is the actual trigger that makes school lunchtime so unpleasant for them. I can get curious about whether it is a particular student who is bullying my client and they don't have the communication skills to let me know, so they simply refuse to attend. If they are humming, loudly talking to themselves, or covering their ears, it is a fairly good indication that it is an auditory stimulus that is causing them alarm.

When we consider sensory processing integration through the trauma lens, we must consider early experiences that formed the pathways for that sensory interpretation. Much of our sensory-related abilities are tied to our early relational experiences.

Was there a sensory experience that was traumatic and created a strong negative association with a neutral stimulus? Does the feeling of a leather couch bring back memories of isolation, or of being cold without a blanket to shield the cool touch of the leather? Does the sight of a four-way stop next to a specific gas station evoke a memory of a car accident? Do they then avoid that intersection altogether? Does the smell of a particular brand of household cleaner remind them of the late-night hours when they had to clean an orphanage while waiting for their forever family?

Sensations involving smell often have deep-rooted correlations to memories that keep us safe. A recent publication has identified pathways that connect traumatic smells to anxiety and post-traumatic stress disorder (PTSD). In my own work, I often see strong connections between smell and fear responses rooted in early adversity. Because of this, it is good to consider laundry detergents, cleaning products, substance smell (alcohol, tobacco, marijuana), colognes, and even smells common to places of abuse such as bath products or garage items. In some situations, smell alone can influence where our mental state is on the arousal continuum.

When I graduated OT school, I was told to avoid perfumes and scented hair products. I see the benefit in this generalization and have interacted with people who wear strong scents that made my olfactory receptors cringe. Because of this, I tend to shy away from scented candles and other strong background scents in my own clinic. However, I have an office manager, Judy, who enjoys candles. Judy sometimes uses fragrances in my office because there are often "farm smells" that need to be covered up since I work at a care farm. Even though I prefer not to use candles, in these moments, scented candles can become therapeutic.

I can use the candle to help a child co-regulate through an unpleasant farm scent sensation if needed. We can't uniquely modify the environment for every child. It is unreasonable to try to control the entirety of sensory input. But, with compassion and connection, we can help broaden their sensory tolerances. When we think back to how we integrate and tolerate non-preferred smells, it is often through relationship, distraction, and proprioception. I lean into this along with the understanding that some of the greatest learning happens in the alert zone and when we are challenged. Some of our best relational advances are in the moments of repair. If a client doesn't like the candle, I can say, "Me neither! But Miss Judy loves them, and we want to help make this pleasant for her. (I model empathy.) Because she sure does help us a lot! She even buys those mints you really like. (I find a personal connection for the client.)" I might pinch my nose and invite them to do the same mirrored proprioceptive input that will also block the nasal passage. We can be playful about it. We can talk about how it covers up the llama fart smell if the client is in the obsession-with-farts phase of development.

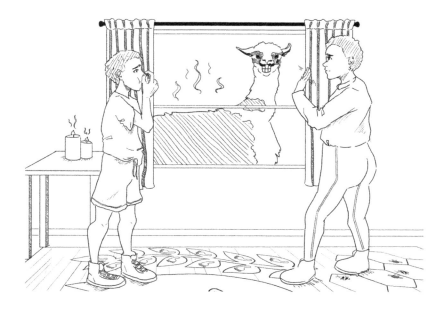

Our relationships can strengthen in adversity. The key (from Dr. Perry's teaching) is mild/moderate stress influence that is patterned and predictable. We can use the mild adversity of an unpleasant scent to co-regulate and teach that we can overcome unpleasant sensations together. As I'm asking them to endure the non-preferred scent, we are engaged in playful purposeful activities. We can be blowing bubbles, playing in the Lycra cloud, or swinging in a swing. These activities are all great sensory distractions. The powerfully regulating vestibular sense is a great override for other sensations. Parents often pick a child up and swing them around joyfully as a distraction when the child is over-focused on something that isn't best for them to engage in. When we are trying to encourage a child to engage, we playfully change our position to get below their eye level so that their own head moves and engages the vestibular system. We shake our heads to "clear our mind." We move our head to regulate because the vestibular system is tied so intimately to our arousal levels and other sensations.

If they are not ready for this co-regulation yet, I can simply blow out the candle and open a window. But then we are dealing with the farm smell. As with most things in life, we find ways to make the best of the situation...together.

As I begin to assess the sensory system, I'm looking at more than the "preferences." I find simple ways to get me wondering what direction to take my treatment plan. While there are standardized tests that give full evaluative outcomes, I often find simple checklists to be quick and easy, leading me to some interesting questions. Personally, I did not pursue the certification for the more advanced sensory evaluations because of cost and time considerations not fitting with the goals of my small private practice. However, if someone seems to be very sensory involved, I have suggested they receive these evaluations at a larger local clinic where the therapists are certified in these evaluations.

In my clinic, I created a sensory response checklist that asks the caregiver or client to rate if certain sensational experiences help them feel safe and calm or more anxious and alert. If my client is often engaging in the activating activities, my treatment and assessment lean towards the assumption that their nervous system is in a higher arousal state than the baseline calm from the state-dependent continuum. I will match their rhythm and desire for more activating activities while I work to bring in more proprioceptive rhythm and calm to their treatment sessions. If my client is fearful of the alerting activities and often engages in the more calming sensational activities, their nervous system may still be in a higher arousal state, but I get curious about whether they are more fearful of sensations that don't integrate well for them. My treatment for these clients tends to move towards slow therapeutic engagement with plenty of felt-safety parameters to experience a wider variety of external sensations. I also tend to bring in more specific protocols that might influence a sensory system such as the auditory, tactile, or vestibular systems more individually and intentionally.

A copy of the following pages, marked with ✶, can be downloaded from www.jkp.com/catalogue/book/9781839975004.

Trauma Lens Sensory Activity Response Checklist from Marti Smith, OTR/L

As you work through these activities, check if the activity brings the client pleasure or restful calm, feels neutral, or makes them anxious or fearful. Make notes if you are not sure. The notes column is for clarity and included with the intention of personalization. It may be helpful to indicate in the notes column which sensory activities may have been influenced by previous trauma or adversity. The goal of this checklist is to assist the person filling it out to identify activities that are dependent upon integration of the various senses. This list is intended for curiosity purposes and to help identify sensory-based patterns. It is not meant to diagnose. It is recommended that the user find a knowledgeable occupational therapist to assist them with interpretation.

When looking for the patterns, be curious. Consider the following:

- Activities that could be influenced by trauma or adversity are marked with a "T." Whether something is perceived as traumatic is incredibly personal and individual. The notes column is for clarification if needed.

- Activities usually involving relationships are marked with an "R." Sometimes it isn't the sensation, but rather the proximity and involvement of other people that might cause decreased sensory capacity. For some individuals, the complexity of being in relationship with others decreases their capacity to engage in sensory activities. For others, adding predictability, routine, perceived control, or relational support can increase their capacity for these activities. If there is a lot of relational activity strength, treatment might be reinforced by relational influence. If relational activity is highly deficient, it may be beneficial to address relational security first, because co-regulation and relationship are the heart of the human sensory experience.

- When a client enjoys a lot of typically alerting stimuli, I look for patterns in the type of sensation they are seeking most. I wonder if they are looking for more information from that sense in order to feel safe. Or I wonder if their body has difficulty perceiving or integrating it. My treatment for these individuals could look like isolating the activity and helping them safely explore the sensation with more intensity.

- When a client is more anxious or fearful, I help them avoid the intensity of these sensations initially and work to incorporate more preferred sensations to help them integrate the most fearful sensations. I pair preferred and non-preferred sensations and work intentionally to make sure they have felt-safety during this exploration.

- Typically activating and typically calming activities are separated in this checklist. I find it helps to see patterns of felt-safety more easily this way. If a child is fearful of activating activities but is comforted by calming activities, I can lean into the calm activities they seem to like most as I pair them to expand their capacity for the more alerting activities. If they enjoy the activating activities more than the calming activities, I am curious about whether they feel safer when sensations are a bit more chaotic and thus match early childhood experiences that were influenced by trauma or adversity.

★

Typically activating types of sensory activities

	Vestibular activities	Calm or enjoyable	Neutral	Anxious or fearful	Notes
R	Non-rhythmic quick movement interactions (fighting, sport moves)				
	Non-rhythmic spinning				
	Running around aimlessly				
	Constantly moving when social construct is to be still				
	Moving playground equipment (swinging, climbing, spinning)				
	Feet not touching the floor				
	Movement that signals nausea				

	Auditory activities	Calm or enjoyable	Neutral	Anxious or fearful	Notes
R	Loud voices of others				Code as fearful if the client thinks people are yelling when others don't
R T	Yelling and loud arguing/disagreements				
R	Crowds such as cafeteria or grocery stores				Could also be smell sensitivity
R	Whispering				
R	Lip smacking, chewing				

		Calm or enjoyable	Neutral	Anxious or fearful	Notes
R	Coughing				
	Loud music				
	Rap/highly rhythmic music/fast-tempo music				This also provides a proprioceptive sensation
T	Sudden sounds such as alarms (even quiet ones) or outside traffic				
	High pitches such as babies crying or puppies barking				
T	Helicopters, planes, fireworks				

	Smell activities	Calm or enjoyable	Neutral	Anxious or fearful	Notes
R T	Perceived negative smells that remind them of individuals				Cologne can be a big fear response smell for some people
R	Smells of others (body odor)				
R T	Tobacco, drugs, alcohol				
R	Bodily fluids				
T	Smells most people find offensive (gas, onion, smoke)				
T	Unfamiliar smells				
T	Bathroom smells				Specify if cleaner or body odors
	Food smells that client doesn't like				

★

	Vision activities	Calm or enjoyable	Neutral	Anxious or fearful	Notes
R	Eye contact				
RT	Eyes looking around entire room (seeking familiarity/exits/safety)				Room scanning, especially for exits, can signal lack of felt-safety
R	Eye–hand-reliant games (ball catch, racket games)				
	Sunlight or bright lights				
	Spinning, flashing, or pulsing lights				Rhythmic lights can have a calming effect, even when they appear stimulating
	Two-dimensional screens				
	Cluttered backgrounds				
	Viewing items in the periphery				
	Looking left to right				
T	Dim light in unsafe areas such as a dark alleyway				Code as fearful if the client is unable to "talk themselves through the situation"

	Taste activities	Calm or enjoyable	Neutral	Anxious or fearful	Notes
	Intense flavors (spicy, garlic, onion, dark chocolate, sour, very salty, peppermint)				
	Foods that scatter in the mouth (carrots, kale, some meats)				
	Foods that scatter are difficult to motor plan				

	Fizzy drinks Fizzy drinks also provide tactile sensory input				
	Cold or hot food Temperatures provide more sensory input				
	Toothpaste, toothbrushing				
	Eating non-food items				

	Proprioceptive activities	Calm or enjoyable	Neutral	Anxious or fearful	Notes
RT	Playful wrestling Mutual wrestling can be alerting because it is non-rhythmic; however, an end result can often be increased serotonin and post relaxation				
	Touches the wall or boundaries in a room The tactile sense can compensate for poor proprioceptive awareness				
	Sheets tucked tightly in bed				
	Chairs that are hard to get out of (bean bags, lots of cushions)				
T	Physical aggression				Code as fearful only if fear of aggression prevents engaging in daily activities and routines

★

	Interoceptive activities	Calm or enjoyable	Neutral	Anxious or fearful	Notes
R	Expressing feelings of anger and disgust				
	Constipation				
T	Pain response				Code calm if client engages in self-injurious behavior; neutral if they do not

	Tactile activities	Calm or enjoyable	Neutral	Anxious or fearful	Notes
R	Wearing "fancy" (uncomfortable) clothing				Does conforming to social norms override sense of comfort?
R T	Light touch non-sensual massage				
R T	Unexpected touch				
R T	Crowds where people might bump into the client				
R T	Sexual touch, intimacy				Code neutral if client isn't sexually active
	Paint or other wet textures on hands				
	Tags in clothes				
	Wearing loose clothes				
	Showers				Showers can be felt as light touch

★

		Calm or enjoyable	Neutral	Anxious or fearful	Notes
	Uneven textures (moving from sidewalk to grass or clothing with mixed fabrics)				
	Being barefoot				
	Washing face				
	Washing hands				Could be more concerned with germs than tactile sensations
	Bumpy foods (oatmeal or casserole)				
	Touches everything in environment (hand on wall when walking, feels every shirt in the store, runs fingers through other's hair without asking first)				
	Washing dishes				
T	Injections, medical procedures (nasal swab)				
	Wanting to be without clothing				

	Non-specific sensory system activities	Calm or enjoyable	Neutral	Anxious or fearful	Notes
R	Rhythmic rituals (drum circles, group dance)				
R	Large social gatherings				
R	Amusement rides				
T	Scary experiences such as horror films, Halloween events, suspenseful movies				

★

Typically calming types of sensory activities

	Vestibular activities	Calm or enjoyable	Neutral	Anxious or fearful	Notes
R	Rhythmic dancing				
R	Rhythmic sports (tennis, skateboarding, swimming, cheerleading)				
	Rhythmic spinning				
T	Riding in a car				

	Auditory activities	Calm or enjoyable	Neutral	Anxious or fearful	Notes
R T	Deep voices				
R	Their own loud voice				
	Nature sounds				
T	Quiet				
	Hums more than others				
T	Covers ears				
	Background noise				
	Slow-tempo music				
	Caregiver lullaby				

★

	Smell activities	Calm or enjoyable	Neutral	Anxious or fearful	Notes
R	Smells of others that are pleasant and familiar				
R	Positive smells that remind them of individuals (Grandma's special bread)				
	Own body smells				
	Food smells that they like				
	Familiar smells				

	Vision activities	Calm or enjoyable	Neutral	Anxious or fearful	Notes
R	Reading				Reading can be a normalized way to dissociate
	Wearing a ball cap or hoodie				Blocking vision sends a normative "I'm not interested in being social" signal
T	Dark or dimly lit spaces that feel safe (movie theater, bedroom)				Some individuals with poor proprioception rely on vision to compensate and may avoid dark spaces for fear of not knowing where they are
	Focal vision—looking intently at one thing positioned at the individual's midline				
	Looking up and down				Looking up facilitates a dissociative response

★

	Taste activities	Calm or enjoyable	Neutral	Anxious or fearful	Notes
R T	Familiar familial/heritage foods				
R	Foods eaten with friends or family				Score "seeks" if child eats more in social context and "avoids" if they eat less in social situations
	Mild flavors (vanilla, milk chocolate, apple)				
	Foods that stick together when wet (chicken nuggets, goldfish crackers, animal crackers, bread)				Sticky foods are easier to swallow; this could also be an oral motor issue
	Milky or creamy drinks				
	Cold or hot food Temperatures provide more sensory input				
	Warm or tepid food				

	Proprioceptive activities	Calm or enjoyable	Neutral	Anxious or fearful	Notes
R T	Hugs				
R	Heavy clothing (layers, weighted vests, heavy sweatshirts)				
R	Rhythmic jumping, stomping, hopping side by side				

		Calm or enjoyable	Neutral	Anxious or fearful	Notes
R	Walking or running side by side				
R T	Massage (not light touch)				
R	Weighted cushions, weighted blankets				
	Walking on toes				
	A smaller foot surface area increases pressure and signal strength of sensation				
	Rhythmic, repetitive stimulation involving force (chewing gum, clicking a pen, tapping a leg, picking scabs, pulling hair)				
	Crashes and bumps into things forcefully				
	Eating chewy foods (breads, pastas, chewy candy, cheese)				

Interoceptive activities	Calm or enjoyable	Neutral	Anxious or fearful	Notes
R T Expressing feelings of acceptance, love, and gratitude				
Breathing in and out slowly and deeply				
Regular bowel movements				
Comfortable body temperature				

★

	Tactile activities	Calm or enjoyable	Neutral	Anxious or fearful	Notes
R T	Hugs for comfort				
R T	Holding hands				
R	Having hair brushed				
R T	Non-sexual touch, intimacy				
	Brushing own hair				
	Wearing comfy clothes				
	Wearing tight clothes				
	Season-appropriate clothes				
	Baths				
	Smooth foods				
	Crunchy foods				

With these simplistic checklists, I'm looking for patterns within the systems. Does the child appear to be either calm or fearful in most areas? Is it a mix? I rarely have a child who is checked in only one column. When we understand how the nervous system perceives and interprets these stimuli based on "Is it safe for me or not with consideration of my past experiences?" we can better understand how to calm or stimulate the system to optimize functional outcomes.

Sometimes, the checklist gives us an indication of a weaker sensory system that is being compensated by another system. For example, if a child is auditorily fearful, they may enhance input to the tactile system as they attempt to navigate their surroundings. I see a lot of children who overly rely on the visual system; when it is taken away, they have a really hard time knowing where they are in relation to their surroundings. This may be why they have to feel their way down a dark hallway, or they get overly anxious without a night light. A child who moves towards a lot of visual sensations and has difficulty knowing where they are in relation to other people and objects may need therapeutic input to the proprioceptive system, such as adding a weighted garment or playing in a crash pad. A favorite proprioceptive activity in my therapy room is to jump on a trampoline with their eyes closed while I hold their hands and give extra auditory instruction to assist with their felt-safety.

These checklists provide an opportunity to be curious, especially when there seems to be "no pattern." When I see check marks that appear random, I look for the relationship. Literally. I get curious if the things they code fearful have to do with people. If they avoid the lunchroom, recess, bathing, and seek loud music, hoodies, and dark spaces, I wonder if they are actually trying to protect themselves from human interaction. When we are hurt by humans, our nervous system works to protect us from humans. I get curious if there seem to be patterns between the sense categories. If they avoid textures but seek smell and taste, do they have difficulty processing textures (maybe an oral motor area to investigate)? Are they looking for more taste and smell because they don't "feel" their food appropriately? What other ways do these tendencies seem to connect?

I look for discrepancies within environments. If Mom fills out an entirely different form than school, Dad, or the child (if old enough),

I wonder if the child feels most comfortable expressing their true feelings with Mom. Are they in the dissociative/possum side of the arousal continuum? Are they exhibiting robotic compliance in other settings, but Mom gets to see their "true self"? Are they holding it together for every other area and falling apart at home? Are their tendencies more polar at school, where maybe they are more challenged and overwhelmed? Understanding how a child's sensory integration is state dependent helps us to know how they perceive things in different environments that will push them into different states of arousal. It can also give me clues about the parent's sensory preferences. If Dad scores completely differently than other settings, I get curious about the lens through which he interprets sensory expression and preferences. For a father who tends to hold feelings inside and does not enjoy loud noises, a high-pitched, easily excited little girl is going to send signals of alarm to Dad's nervous system. Maybe I need to help Dad see what is "normal" and how we can work together to meet his child's sensory-seeking needs in a way that keeps his own nervous system calm. We educate Dad that he doesn't always need to be calm. Sometimes, playful activity is best engaged in within the alert stage of the continuum. We find songs Dad enjoys where they can scream out the words together. Because when the screaming is patterned and predictable, it will lower the perceived stress for Dad, but still meet the need for the child to scream. While there is no single "magic cure" for expanding sensory capacity, that curiosity and therapeutic process is magical as we watch families build empathy and compassion for differing sensory preferences and capacities.

Suggestions for therapeutic activities that help with **sensory processing** taken from the KALMAR app:

- Chewing gum, music, swimming, and other **sensory-rich activities** can help a child better understand their sensory world through co-experience with a trusted and loving caregiver.

- Exercise with **proprioceptive emphasis** (crash and bump) engages the proprioceptive system, which can help activate the cortex to aid in discrimination tasks.

- **Forward flexion and midline activities** tend to anatomically calm the body while extension and moving away from midline tend to alert the body.

- Use **rhythm** to calm and non-rhythm to alert.

- **Modify the physical environment** for support with an emphasis on sensory mindfulness. Ask the individual what they prefer in regard to environmental sensations and work to match their preferences during therapeutic activities. Working in dimmed light, adding a diffuser, or playing their favorite song in the background is a great way to help a client know they are "seen" and valued.

CHAPTER 5

• • • •

The Limbic Area

The limbic area is the hub that connects the sensational feelings to the emotions and determines how they are stored as memories. This area of the brain includes, among other structures, the thalamus, hypothalamus, amygdala, and hippocampus. I like to refer to the limbic area as the "kill me or not" center. This is the customs area where information is sorted and tagged for future reference as safe or unsafe. Based on the conclusion of this sorting analysis, these structures then connect with other brain structures for an adaptive response. Some information (such as pain, light touch, and temperature) is assessed to be an immediate threat. These sensations travel up the spinal cord to parts of the autonomic nervous system that provide immediate response to keep us safe. These parts include the cerebellum along with the somatic nervous system, including the motor cortex for quick muscle movements to move us to safety and the memory centers to remember to not get in that unsafe situation again. So when we experience these fearful sensations, there is very little "thought" about how we initially respond. I'm quick to remind caregivers and clients that when an individual struggles with integration of these sensations, they are neurologically wired to move to protective mode. It is not an intentional, manipulative, or personal response. It is the result of their unconscious neurobiology attempting to put their body into a perceived state of safety. Often, the *why* behind a behavior is simply a responsive moving away from a threat or towards something that is perceived as safe.

The **thalamus** transmits 98 percent of sensory information to the cortex, including vision, taste, touch, and balance. It is a limbic structure that is part of the higher order of the brain where specific sensory discriminative stimuli (except for smell) land and is quickly (nanoseconds) assessed. The thalamus also plays a role in sleep, wakefulness, consciousness, learning, and memory. When I think of limbic structures, the thalamus is one of the first to come to mind. This is because it is a major hub that connects so many neurological processes within this limbic system.

The **hypothalamus** has been called the heart of the brain. It is involved with releasing hormones, controlling appetite, maintaining physiological cycles such as heart rate and sleep, sexual behavior, and regulating emotional responses and body temperature. Dopamine (feel-good hormone) and corticotropin (stress hormone) are created in the hypothalamus. If your hypothalamus is not working optimally, it's difficult to "feel" good. It also plays an important role in addiction, reward, and mood. The hypothalamus is also integral to the processing of mobilization and immobilization due to the nociceptive cues of safety or threat.

The **amygdala** was once believed to be the primary center for processing fear, but recent research has suggested that basic sensory processing detects potential threats, and the amygdala contributes to the emotional tone that builds the emotion of fear from the affect of threat. In particular, the olfactory system is a potentially significant player. This is intriguing because the olfactory sense stands alone among the cranial nerves in that it does not initially pass through the thalamus and thus, the information is processed directly and quickly, and any olfactory-based threat trigger quickly mobilizes a response.

While it's possible that the amygdala may not be the exclusive fear center, it remains crucial in the complex landscape of human affective and emotional experiencing. The amygdala is involved in fear responses, the perception of intense emotions like anger and sadness, and the regulation of our reactions to aggression. Additionally, it plays a pivotal role in the encoding of memories related to stressful events. Unlike its limbic system neighbor, the hippocampus, which is shut down in memory encoding during extreme stress, the amygdala helps to hold threat memories for future reference. These memories serve as valuable tools, equipping us to better avoid or escape similar situations if they recur in the future

The **hippocampus** is further specialized in emotional memory consolidation, learning, emotional responses, and spatial navigation. It takes in the information, registers it, and temporarily stores it to be filed in long-term memory.

When our limbic system is activated as we move towards terror on our arousal continuum, our arousal and emotional self-regulation become deficient. We become "overly emotional" because we are feeling too many things without integrating them. Or we become disconnected relationally because the structures that are supposed to integrate and sort these feelings out are having a difficult time making sense of the senses and situations, so we "dial down" our response to them. Just as difficulty in the cerebellum and brainstem throws off our internal rhythms, difficulty in the limbic system can throw off our emotions, interoception, sleep, appetite, and memory. The limbic system provides the mood or tone for our mental state.

As we view the limbic system through the lens of trauma and relationships, we can see how complex it is to self-regulate and relate to others. Without a caring, connected caregiver to model and help us unpack our emotions and feelings as we relate to them, we are left with no scaffolding or support for what that even looks like. When our memories make sensory connections that code benign daily-life sensations as fearful daily-life sensations, it makes it difficult to navigate even familiar people and places. When the unknown is introduced, there is simply too much risk of those memories coding so many things as fear. As we seek to become trauma responsive, we must always be considering how someone's sensory perceptions and preferences are intricately connected to their past experiences. We must also remember that these connections are hard-wired into the subconscious and very emotional limbic system structures.

Functions that are mediated in the limbic system that occupational therapists can influence include:

- emotions

- matching the regulatory state of the environment and social cues

- relating to others

- interoception as it modulates feelings and body sensations.

Emotions

My friend and Simple Sparrow Care Farm co-founder, Jamie Tanner, once said, "That child has big feelings" as she witnessed a child yelp and cry hysterically when they stubbed their toe. As she said this, I realized how appropriate that description was for so many of the individuals I work with. They feel things "big" and they express them "big." Some clients are told via words and actions very early in life that they don't have value, or their emotions don't matter until those emotions are very "big." They may not have been cared for unless their words and actions were loud enough to be heard. If their reactions weren't big, they were not noticed.

Many of my clients find me because their reactions tend to be described as intense, over-exaggerated, or not matching the social situation. When we consider how the limbic system structures assess sensory stimulation as "kill me or not," we can consider that these big feelings are biological and not intentional. If the memory centers consider sensory input to be a threat, the reaction is initiated before the planes fly from that thalamus hub to the prefrontal cortex for inhibition and reasoning.

One thing I find helpful is to consider that we will always have a first thought. Our first thought often gets out before the structures that inhibit the fear response are activated. With time and practice, we can influence and even change our first thoughts. But, until we know better, we will sometimes have a first thought that doesn't align with our desires. As adults, we have more experience and capacity to not always express those first thoughts, and the wisdom to know our first thought may not be true. I once had a friend joke that when her husband is more than 30 minutes late, she begins to plan her life as a widow. With each passing minute, her brain begins to move along the arousal continuum unless she is able to call him and prove her first thoughts wrong with the concrete data of his assuring voice. She doesn't actually start planning his funeral, but the situational anxiety highlights her fear of him being in a car accident. This fear leads her to have thoughts that do not align with her normal thinking. But she is able to have second thoughts of assuring herself there are many reasons he could be late. Maybe his car was needing gas, or she forgot about an errand or extra meeting. With our clients, it is helpful to allow them to express those first thoughts without judgment and then help them to recognize ways those thoughts are not true when they are ready.

I try to make my therapy room a place of non-judgment. When I have clients with different skin colors or outward expression of gender, I can sometimes sense a distrust that I don't mirror them in many ways physically. For these clients, I recognize that I need to demonstrate safety, inclusion, and acceptance to them. I do this by being curious and open to dialogue. Compliments on specifics such as hair or clothing, or even noticing something as they walk in the door—"Oh, your hair reminds me of (insert someone relatable to the client here). Did they influence your style?"—can go a long way to acknowledge our differences with respect. I can also be more open-ended, such as "I really like that pattern on your tattoo. Was it inspired by something?" I might compliment their outfit and ask where they like to shop for clothing items. This can be an indication that this very white and comfortably styled middle-aged cis normal person about to dig into their personal business is at least interested in who they truly are. I see my clients as individuals and strive to let them know their unwavering value in my eyes, regardless of age, background, or ability. I continue to work through my own journey, and I want them to know their emotions, beliefs, and values are welcome in my space, even if they are different from mine. Current neuroscience supports the need to express our felt-senses of self. I have secure attachments outside of my therapy room walls and ways to cope with my own emotions that help me have strong practiced ways of remaining in my frontal cortex in the moment, even when the person I need to co-regulate may not have full access to their own.

Some clients I work with experienced abuse or neglect as a child. Some clients are queer in a non-supportive family. They did not have a loving, attuned, compassionate caregiver to help guide them through or even help name their emotions. They did not sit with them and help guide them with support strategies. These clients don't know how to name or even express their feelings. They have very few descriptive words and adjectives to describe them.

Even without the background of intentional abuse or neglect, some caregivers are not able to correctly interpret the cues of the baby, and thus the baby has difficulty knowing how to get their needs met until their feelings are very "big" and the caregiver finally succeeds in calming them on the umpteenth attempt to soothe them. I say this last sentence with deep compassion. Libraries would not be full of baby books if it was easy to interpret the cues of a baby. Being mis-attuned is something that causes many caregivers to feel shame, but it is very common. Disconnection is not imminent when the caregiver continues to seek ways to connect and meet the needs. With each repair, the brain sends signals of attachment that counteract the signals of mis-attunement. Repair can be even more powerful than never having mis-attunement. Repair leads to resilience and the understanding that things cannot be perfect, but I'm still connected to my caregiver who will help me co-regulate until I learn to self-regulate.

As I begin to address the goals related to emotions, I first lean into ways our emotions can be influenced. Once I figure out how to evoke an emotion in a client, we can work together to identify what that emotion is. When we can name it, we can tame it, *if it needs to be tamed*. I am clear with my clients that if an emotion is designed to keep them safe, I don't want to remove it unless they feel safe. If they aren't feeling safe often, that needs to be the first thing I address. If I simply stop the aggression but don't take away the trigger for the aggression, I've only trained this client to dissociate inappropriately. I want to figure out what is making the person aggressive so that I can then work to change the need for that response. For example, if I have a child who hits and kicks every time I put him in a car seat, I don't want to just train him to stop. I want to know why he hates the car seat. Can we change his position in the car from the left side to the right side? Can we try a five-point harness for more stability or a booster for less tactile input? Can we improve his postural stability so that he can hold himself up better and not feel so unsupported in a car? Do we need to not have an unreasonable expectation of stopping at five stores as we are doing morning errands? I remember reading once that three is the errand max. The average toddler falls apart after three errands in a row without a physical movement/creative break. Sometimes we need to match our expectations to the abilities of the child at that moment.

Once I've removed the threat or done a good activity analysis as to the *why* behind the big feelings/emotions, I can begin to build new neural experiences that make them more agreeable. I can use animals to help identify what things influence their mood. Examples would be when a dog wags his tail as he sees us approaching for connection or licks his lips or (gross!) drools when we get ready to feed him. We can talk about how the client responds to similar situations. Sometimes they will match, sometimes they will not. For my potty-obsessed young children, I can be silly about how animals might eat poop and how that would be delicious and exciting for them but disgusting and repulsive for us. I can smell different candles or spices from the kitchen, and we can reminisce about memories and emotions we associate with these smells.

When we identify how things in our environment make us feel, we can explore how we can use our pairing strategy to link sensations together. If I know lemon makes me energized, I can use a lemon cleaner to help me stay focused on cleaning my house. If I know soft music is calming for me, I can play soft music during the last hour before bedtime to set the mood for the nightly routine. If I can understand that a warm bath calms me, I can exchange 30 minutes in the bathtub for the 30 minutes of scrolling doomsday news. Or, if I can see how my child calms when he runs and alerts when he chews peppermint gum, I can experiment with those paired sensations when the task at hand requires calm but my child is needing to alert. What would happen if I gave him peppermint gum and ran a lap around the house? If choking is a risk, I could rub peppermint scented (skin safe) product on his wrist instead of putting gum in his mouth.

Giving my clients freedom to understand that emotions keep them safe and are welcome around me helps them begin to discover more information about how their individual body reacts to different sensations. This awareness alone can help them manage these emotions better. Sometimes, when we understand the *why* behind an emotion, it is less overwhelming. When we give our body permission to feel, we can sometimes take the extra 30 seconds to allow our prefrontal cortex to catch up with our second thought before we have big mismatched feelings and emotions.

Suggestions for therapeutic activities that help with **emotions** taken from the KALMAR app:

- Allow for **extra time** to transition between activities. Add rhythm (songs, marching, clapping) between events.

- **Animals are silent confidants**. It is easier to explore emotions with animals than it is with people when an individual experiences trauma with people.

- Find a **variety of sensory experiences** and allow the child to "feel" the sensations. Mirror them, parallel with them. Talk about how you feel and open your curiosity for any reaction they may have that could be the same or different. Remember that no feeling is wrong. "That's remarkable" is a good response when a client says something that is actually really hot is cold. Then add that the water feels cold to you. But do not tell them they are wrong. Exhibit more curiosity than correction.

- **Massage**, when an individual is open to it, can be a great way to discover where they are most tight in their muscles. Once discovered, this can lead to curiosity about if they feel as though their body is holding any tension from unexpressed emotions.

- **"Powerfully You"** (www.powerfullyyou.org) is a curriculum that helps guide individuals through their emotions in a trauma-responsive, respectful, relevant, and engaging way.

Matching the regulatory state of the environment and social cues

Matching the regulatory state of the environment and social cues requires knowing what the social norms are and being able to understand subtle non-verbal nuances. If my client is able to move independently between states of calm and alert but goes immediately into alarm or fear when in the presence of a group, they may have a difficult time understanding social norms or cues. These clients tend to be diagnosed as oppositional, defiant, antisocial, or even bipolar.

As an aside, I dislike seeing children under the age of 12 diagnosed with personality disorders. From a personal perspective, I was a hot mess express as a young kid. That express train could have easily pulled into a dysfunction junction and loaded up with all kinds of labels I'm glad I don't have on record today. I'm a vastly different person than I was in my teens. I'm guessing many of the readers of this book feel the same way. How can we possibly label so many kids with a diagnosis from the personality categories before the part of the brain that influences our personality is even developed?

A hundred years ago, there were aunties and grannies as neighbors who would spend time with children to teach them how to get along with others and learn a family trade. While the ideal caregiving situation is four older caregivers (some siblings) to one child, we boast when our preschools have a staff ratio of two adults to 15 toddlers. Our families are geographically moving apart, and our neighbors are online instead of outdoors. An unfortunate trend that I am noticing, especially after the impact of Covid isolation, is that children are expected to understand social norms without a caregiver walking alongside them to teach them. With parents trying to work from home, children are being told to go into another room and fend for themselves. Parents are working to put food on the table and the child's physical needs are being met. Maybe the exhausted parent is even able to read them a bedtime story at night and is as connected as possible when they are not working. But the reality of Covid disconnection remains. Many children born between 2019 and 2022+ do not have the needed practice of large social gatherings to be able to read the room and understand societal expectations. If we want them to be successful in these areas, we must take the time to teach them.

When a child's activation of alertness doesn't match the societal expectation, we must first ask if the expectation is too high and then assess if the child even knows what is expected. If it is not an awareness or developmental appropriateness issue, I, as the occupational therapist, go back to activity analysis. What is causing the problem? I think through the brain sequence and hub structures. Does this child feel safe? Are their biological needs met? Is there a supportive caregiver available to help them co-regulate? Is the sensory environment set up in a way that this person is able to integrate the sensations they are taking in? Do they have internal motivation to be a part of the group? Do they understand the purpose of the group and how they fit in?

In my therapy space, I make Social Stories (Gray, 2000) of expectations and we practice them in a supportive environment. We role-play and engage in "what if" scenarios. I give lots of positive and non-judgmental "noticing" of how they are or are not matching the social cues of the environment or situation. A therapeutic activity example is using horse-assisted role play in a school bully simulation. During our session, I allow the therapy horse to get too close and invade my client's personal space. Then I model and teach the child to push the horse away physically and verbally. We talk about how we can use force to keep our bodies safe and sometimes we need to be more assertive with others who get too close in our personal bubbles. Large animals are beneficial for modeling social interactions. The animal removes the pressure of the human relationship, and large dogs and horses can be felt with the entire body for more cueing on parallel interaction. When you are riding a horse, you have no option but to go at the pace of the horse. If you get too rough with a dog, they will let you know. If the dog is resting but the child comes in with heightened energy, the dog will likely move away or disengage at first. If the dog is excited and the child is too low-energy/has low activation, the dog will do playful things to engage the child. Dogs are eager to repair and thus encourage the re-dos that help clients practice new strategies of engaging. This is yet another reason I love using animals in my therapy sessions.

Another therapeutic activity example is to engage siblings in a play activity that the caregiver has told me will lead to an argument. As I watch the interactions unfold, I can give each sibling cues to read the body language of the other sibling. Sometimes, the reaction is to laugh in the moment and tease one another. Other times, they may escalate into an actual argument in the session. This can be normal for the first few practices. I often see a shift in the third or fourth interaction. As I get better at reading the cues of the children, I get better at helping them read the cues of one another. I use fun activities and reinforcements. I find ways to use Lycra where it takes two people to be successful and it's motivating for both to engage. There are several "team-building exercises" on Pinterest that fuel my ideas. I get better buy-in and success when I can tailor the activity to the siblings and have their input before we get started. A favorite is simply drumming in turn. Both siblings are in a net swing next to each other. Each sibling picks a drum and can choose their own beat until the timer goes off. While one is drumming, I am physically moving the swing of the other sibling to match the playing sibling's beat. Then they get to take turns. Matching the social context takes time and practice.

When I have a child who is exhibiting too much energy for the situational context, I become curious about why their nervous system appears to be so activated. Often, the increased movement is due to a base arousal state that has been tipped towards the fear state. I imagine this child is trying to experience more sensory information as their limbic system is trying to assess and respond to their surroundings. Once again, I lean into rhythm. If the movements and activity appear to have a rhythmic pattern, it tells me that the nervous system is leaning into the cerebellum and brainstem, looking to calm itself by taking in more rhythmic and proprioceptive information. If the movements of the child appear to be arhythmic, it tells me that the nervous system is having difficulty making sense of the information and is therefore looking for more sensory stimulation as a way of gaining more cues in regard to safety.

Once I assess the rhythmicity of the child's activity and movement, I attempt to match their rhythm to tip them into co-regulation with me. While I'm doing this, I'm looking for signs of felt-safety. I'm assessing the environment for possible threat activators for them. If I'm talking, I'm conscious of my speaking rate, pitch, and tone. I'm matching the timing of my inhalations to their breath. I'm mirroring body positions in very subtle, respectful, and non-teasing ways in an attempt to engage the mirror neurons to help them get in sync with my activation levels. While I maintain my calm state of mind, I may purposefully activate my body and affect to match their alert state before I attempt to influence their regulatory state—*with* mine. In the same way, I use rhythm in the musical fast/slow game to influence movement patterns, and to influence my client's state of arousal to match the situation and social environments. Because, in order to calm the limbic system, we must first support the lower hierarchical connections within the cerebellum.

Suggestions for therapeutic activities that help with **matching the regulatory state of the environment and social cues** taken from the KALMAR app:

- **Match energy** but not dysregulation. When I work with Robyn, we often bounce ideas around about how to physically match the tempo of a situation in order to connect, but without escalating the situation. If someone is pacing the room and stomping around, you may rock back and forth in a chair in the room to their cadence. But you don't stomp and yell back at them. Or, if they run up to you with a cut on their finger, you respond at the same increased vocal tone as you tell them you are getting a Band-Aid. But you don't ignore them or scold them for how the cut occurred.

- **Adjust expectations** and raise compassion when an individual needs more support with social situations. Experiencing trauma or adversity can code the nervous system to feel threats when things are unpredictable. Allowing compassion in the moment opens the door for conversations about correction, if truly needed, at a later date. Often, if we can adjust our own expectations, we do not need correction.

- **Animals** can be used for emotional support and assistance in accessing environments. When an individual has difficulty with over-stimulating environments, the animal can help calm with a co-regulatory affect, heartbeat, and petting of their fur. Animals also provide a point of interest with conversations when an individual struggles with what to talk about in social situations.

- **Mirror** the client and match your actions to be parallel with them. You may discover something when you can "see" and "feel" their perspective from a different vantage point.

- **Weighted items** are a great way to provide proprioceptive input to an individual's nervous system to help calm them, so they are better able to access their cortical thinking brain during perceived stressful situations.

Relating to others

Once we can relate to ourselves through understanding our own emotions, we can begin to relate to others. Once we are individually feeling safe, we look to our community to be safe with us. This section correlates with the idea that hurt people hurt people, and we learn how to have healthy relationships by *having* healthy relationships. My training material as a TBRI practitioner highlights how our early experiences in the care of our early primary caregivers influence our future attachment styles and capacity to care for and relate to others. If we don't have those thousands of attachment moments where we feel safe and secure in the arms of someone else, safety will be something we continue to seek in maladaptive ways. We may seek inappropriate touch. We may assume people think the worst of us and therefore we hide our best selves. We may desperately want to be with other people but then push them away, not knowing how to actually relate to them. When a client tells me that they want to increase a child's ability to be respectful, I remind them that feeling respected fosters respect. It is difficult to have empathy or understand the perspective of another person if we do not have the same experience ourselves.

When my client has difficulty relating to others, I start with working on self-esteem and understanding who they are as a valued individual. We do collages, vision boards, and simply discussion on what things bring us joy, what things frustrate or scare us, and what we think we are successful with. Most of my clients have plenty of practice with negative self-talk and failure. I try to reframe failure as a good data point for them and work on redirecting the negative self-talk. I validate it in the sense that all feelings are welcome, valued, and explored with curiosity in my therapy space. But I try to counter negativity with positivity, without being dismissive. If a child tells me he isn't good at school and has the low grades to support that, I'm not going to tell him he's smart or say at least he's good at sports. Instead, I'll lean in a little and ask if it is something he would like to work on and if there are ways we can work as a team to support him. Does he need to figure out a good sensory space and strategy for homework? Do we need to work on some eye tracking to read the classroom board or follow the math layouts? Do we need to advocate for a water bottle or frequent movement breaks? I become curious about ways to support them in working towards their potential.

Brendan McCane, OTR, is an occupational therapist colleague who once told me that a common goal for him is to figure out what brings a client joy. That discussion really impacted me. I think of it in tandem with a saying from my childhood—"If you love what you do, you will never work a day in your life." A personal goal for me is to bring joy to as many situations as possible. Life is full of difficulty, trauma, and challenge. If we are going to be successful at the roller coaster of life, we need to buffer those with intentionally finding ways to bring joy to situations, even if it is temporary. Our neurons sometimes just need a quick break to re-calibrate, adjust, and refocus before integrating the more challenging circumstances of being human. Finding what brings my clients joy might be the most powerful goal I ever meet for them. Because, I hope, it will empower them to continue on their journey of life, finding joy among the inherent challenges that life brings.

For humans, joy is meant to be shared. Most joyful moments and experiences involve other humans. For our clients who struggle with relationships, joy is less frequent. If I'm to help them find joy, I need to help them relate to others. This is not an easy task. Humans are complex, and while we desire to have relationships, we have a lot of personal biases that push people away. Our nervous system is a confusing dyad of being fearful of new or different people while simultaneously desiring intimacy. Since the recording of history, humans have always been the biggest threat to other humans. Modern society further complicates this. For hundreds of years, our social circles were very small and likely included people who shared our very DNA and thus heavily mirrored our own appearances. With advancements in travel, migration, and opening up new opportunities to have children with people who don't look just like us, our foundational biases work against us for forming close new relationships. Understanding this brings awareness to why some people have difficulty relating physically to others. We are genetically coded to relate to a very small group of people who look like us and be fearful of the rest. Relating to multiple people who may not look like us must be taught. With repeated positive exposure, we can learn new patterns of positively relating within our beautifully diverse modern-day community.

On the farm, we use animals to be a bridge to relationships. When relating to a human is difficult, sometimes something as small as a rabbit or fish can encourage practice of simple greetings and pleasantries. We learn to care for a living being and then those care skills translate to ourselves and other humans. My daughter once taught me a great medication hack. Feed your cat a treat at the exact same time you take your daily medications. You might forget to take your meds one day. But that cat will give you a very persistent reminder. Because of the non-confrontational way most people engage with animals, it is less confrontational for a cat to remind us of something rather than a well-intended human.

When I don't have access to animals, I work to empower clients with conversational skills. I find ways to help them have something to talk about. I was a magician in college and brought this hobby to my therapy room as a new graduate. I found that I could teach a client a few easy-to-learn magic tricks using accessible materials and it would open the door for social opportunity for them. Cooking can also be a great way to relate. When we teach clients how to cook, we are teaching them how to care not only for their own physical nutrition needs but also the needs of others. Since food is so relationally based, it tends to be an interesting topic to assist our clients to discuss in their desire to relate to others.

Any type of daily activity can be a way to relate to someone. Most people feel more social when they feel valued. Even if someone doesn't like to talk a lot or doesn't know what to say, painting a room together, tending a garden, chopping veggies for an omelet, or washing a family pet together gives the satisfaction of a job well done and the relational benefit of shared success. Even a simple "please pass the carrots/paint/dog shampoo" as we engage in these daily activities can be an open door to communication for some of my clients.

Suggestions for therapeutic activities that help with **relating to others** taken from the KALMAR app:

- **Animal-assisted therapies** are a wonderful way to bridge the gap for clients who experienced relational trauma. By co-caring for an animal, we send the message to the client that we can also care for them. Animals are a great way to teach care for both ourselves and others.

- **Collages** help cue clients to what may interest them. When we are trying to get to know a person, we often ask, "What is your favorite…?" When a client experiences developmental trauma or adversity, they may not fully know what their preferences are. Having a variety of pictures can provide visual cues to help them think about things they enjoy.

- **Dance** can be a wonderful expressive outlet which structures contact and interaction between people in very patterned and predictable ways. When you dance with a partner in formal styles, there is structure and predictability as well as frequent and brief contact with another person. This can help lead to resilience in tolerating someone in proximity.

- **Encouraging eye contact** through play (bubbles, looking at magazines together, or Hedbanz game[1]) or mirroring motor movements with a regulated adult can facilitate brief and playful moments of eye contact which help people feel socially connected.

- **Volunteering** allows an individual to feel a purpose for a greater good which facilitates care for their community.

Interoception as it modulates feelings and body sensations

The limbic structures assess how we "feel" and then release hormones and neurochemicals that catalyst automatic responses for action in our muscles, joints, and organs that prepare us to mobilize or immobilize based on our needs for survival. For example, before we are able to think about something scary that happens quickly, like something scurrying into our path, our heart rate may increase or our muscles

---

1 Hedbanz is a game where players place a card with illustrations of items in a headband that they can't see but other players can. They then ask the other players about what illustration is on their head, in hopes of guessing what is pictured before other players guess what is on their own headbands.

may tense or even activate a jumping response. Interoception isn't something we think about without being intentionally mindful in that moment. Since these physical responses are automatic, it takes practice and intention to be aware of these interoceptive sensations. It is subconscious and its "airport hub" is the insula. If you have recently studied neuroscience, you have likely at least heard of the insula. Having graduated in 1996, I was relieved to find out that the insula and the insular cortex are among the brain structures about which we have gained increased understanding since 2006. If you are seasoned, as I am, I highly recommend a little refresher on this structure. I find it fascinating. It is part of the "Mohawk of self-awareness" that Bessel van der Kolk speaks of in his book *The Body Keeps the Score*. In his book, Bessel discusses how trauma can influence the activation of these self-awareness structures, that are positioned in the superior portion of the brain as if they are creating a figurative mohawk. These structures include the insula, the orbital prefrontal cortex, the medial prefrontal cortex, the anterior cingulate, and the posterior cingulate. In the nervous system's efforts to shut out the pain of the trauma, it actually shuts down feeling oneself as well. This feeling oneself, or interoception, is processed in the lower parts of the insula and then has a higher level of processing in the upper parts of the insula. Through this "Mohawk of self-awareness," these structures connect to give us conscious awareness of our interoceptive signals and experiences.

One of the few things we can consistently control in our bodies is what comes in and what goes out of our digestive tract. Often, when I work with an eating issue or a child who has difficulty with bowel elimination, I find that they are feeling a lack of control in their lives. This is not to say that every case is a control indication or that these clients all can be "healed" by giving them control. But it is often a really good place to start as I consider treatment options. The interoceptive sense is the bridge between the emotional and the physical. In ancient times, it was thought that different organs were responsible for different feelings. Even today, we talk about "gut" feelings, and heart emojis flood our communication to show affection. Our feelings and hormones are directly related to how we view the world. Remembering the arousal continuum, we can see bowels shutting down or activating as we move through that continuum. Our breath and heart rates move up and down as well as we move from calm to terror. Increased activation leads us to sweat or have goosebumps. Our liver and kidneys change secretions as our stress increases or decreases. All these things aid in increasing our chance of survival. When we are calm, the limbic structures send signals to the body that we can connect with others and feel joy, love, and excitement. When we are feeling threatened, we shut down with sadness, anxiety, or anger.

When we don't understand the emotions, we can miss our body cues. Because the body has similar reactions for different feelings. Like our air traffic patterns, we look for patterns to give us a better understanding of how we truly feel. Anger and anxiety can both lead to elevated heart rate and increased bowel movements. Joy, love, and excitement can do the same. I've had "butterflies in my stomach" for both anxiety and excitement about a happy surprise. With anxiety, the butterflies may have accompanied lethargy, while the happy surprise made my muscles feel energized. When we are able to explore these associations within an environment of felt-safety, we can help our clients see these subtle differences in the patterns. I have found the curriculum "Powerfully You" to be incredibly helpful with helping my clients explore and identify their own sense of interoception.

Our emotional awareness can also be learned from our interpersonal relations. There are self-help books and podcasts about what love feels like. How do we know if someone loves us back? How do we know what love really is? If we don't understand the sensations of our own bodies, we can easily fall into abusive relationships where someone *tells* us that they love us. But they don't *show* us. But if we have no understanding of what it should *feel* like, it is difficult to sort all of that out. When we don't understand how we feel, it is difficult to understand how others feel about us. Much of our interoception is directly related to how we feel about how others feel about us. We get anxious with interpersonal conflict, perceived or real. When we are in a healthy connected relationship, we feel joy in the presence of others who are joyful with us.

I help clients explore their interoception from the outside in. Just as I focus on the gross motor before fine motor and the proximal stability before the distal mobility, I move from the outside in with interoceptive awareness. I do this because I have a more objective understanding of what they are experiencing on the outside. I can see it. Often, I'm the one influencing it. Skin is our largest organ. It's easily accessible once I have gained the trust of my client. I can practice something feeling squishy in their fingers to give them a reference for something feeling squishy in their tummy. Even the experience of comparing a hard billiards ball with a soft squishy marshmallow can give context and language to a bowel movement. When I use a vibratory tool and dial it between fast and slow, I can relate that to heart rates. When we have concrete sensation awareness outside, we can begin to relate to our internal sensations.

To increase interoception, I use therapeutic activities that utilize Lycra, tactile sensation play, cooking, nature walks, animal-assisted therapies, and drumming. I even have a playful nickname, the Lycra Princess. I have a trauma tips video on my website (creativetherapies. com), that provides instructions on how to use Lycra in therapeutic ways and have included a section in Chapter 11 about the more technical "how-tos." I even have a Lycra cloud in the entryway of my own home. We are big fans of Lycra in my family. I love how inexpensive, accessible, and versatile it is. It provides a nice proprioceptive "molding" to the body of the client to give them postural support along with therapeutic pressure. I find it an important therapeutic tool to help clients understand how their body relates to the world around them. If you can't feel where you are in the world, it's difficult to know where you are in your body. Lycra provides that extra resistance with their movements and creates pressure on the proprioceptive receptors in both the joints and muscles. Other than diving in water, there is no other modality I am aware of that recreates this calming sensation so vastly and effectively. Lycra builds in an element of safety for many of my clients who have experienced adversity. It provides a womb-like safety of putting the body into a fetal flexion pattern with the constant pressure. It creates a soft barrier between the client and my hand when I need to help facilitate a movement or contact. I ask permission any time I am wanting to make physical contact with my clients. When we have the Lycra barrier, I rarely get a refusal, even from my most sensitive-to-touch clients. I can use the Lycra to provide rhythmic, relational, relevant, respectful, and rewarding stimulation that facilitates integration of interoceptive sensations as we get curious about how the Lycra feels. I may question if it feels soft, smooth, tight, pressurizing, bouncy, stretchy, or cozy. I once had a client tell me it felt "stabilizing," which fit the profile of their loose-feeling joints. If I could only have one therapeutic tool besides my own body, I'm pretty sure I would choose Lycra. For many of my clients, once they can figure out their proprioceptive awareness, so many other therapeutic goals are more easily met.

Tactile sensation play is a wonderful way to playfully engage in new experiences that evoke high emotion. For most clients, playing in shaving cream or running fingers through animal feed is a novel experience. A self-regulated nervous system enjoys novel experiences. But for some of my clients, I need to build in an element of safety and take the experience slow because their nervous system is tipped towards fear because of frequent past fearful experiences. When my client is able to experience this felt-safety, they are better able to safely experience other novel stimulation in the future. They must first build the understanding of "I've touched this texture before, and I did not die. Maybe I'll also survive this encounter." For many, they have never reached the point of "did not die." Because they either avoided or pushed away unfamiliar tactile information. With tactile play, we can talk through textures. We can associate other sensations in tandem. How does that shaving cream or feed mixture smell? Do you have any memories associated with shaving cream or the smell of alfalfa? With shaving cream, I buy the sensitive-skin type so that the smell is not as overwhelming. The bonus is that it is a type of soap that can clean whatever surface you are using it on. I don't limit my shaving cream use location to a table. I might put it over a bumpy tactile ball. I put it into a small bowl and hide little resin animals within the soft white texture. I add liquid watercolors or glitter to change the visual appearance or texture. I encourage playfulness.

Another playful way to explore our bodies relationally is with a clear storage-box lid and dry erase markers. I hold up the clear plastic lid between me and the client. I press it to the tip of my nose and invite them to "decorate my face." It is also a great way to encourage eye contact and connection. One of my very favorite therapy sessions was when I invited a client to decorate my face with shaving cream instead of the markers. He put some on me and then mimicked by putting some on his actual face. It was beautiful. My assistant grabbed a rubber spatula from the kitchen, and we had an impromptu shaving session. This was a child who required a safety rag for all tactile activities. After only 15 minutes of safety and playfulness, he tolerated a soft sticky texture on his face. It was an amazing awakening for his tactile system.

Nature walks are another way to work on interoception because they provide a wide variety and different levels of intensity for sensations. We can walk barefoot on soft sand, pebbles, or grass. Grass in Texas is significantly different from grass in Ohio. Weather can change a session as well. As we think of experiencing known and unknown sensations, weather can provide an unknown backdrop to a known environment. While a rainstorm in a foreign neighborhood could be too much, knowing the terrain and places to duck in for a reprieve from the rain can add an element of unpredictable therapeutic input to the framework of known sensations. A common activity in my own practice is to pause and identify something you "feel." What do you smell? What do you hear? Do you see anything unusual? At Simple Sparrow Care Farm, we try to plant intentional plants that draw both bees and butterflies. Depending on the location on the farm, I can help influence the sensory input that a client experiences. For many, interoceptive awareness can be improved by the small pause that happens while we assess the input. So many of my clients are too busy to notice the bees or the breeze unless it hits the alarming sensation level. Pausing to understand the sensations when they are subtle gives an additional level of understanding of the input. We can identify the sensations and then once again invite our clients to let us know if they enjoy the sensation as we do. We can ask them if it reminds them of something they have experienced before.

I am careful not to tell a client how they feel, and instead allow space for them to tell me how they feel, even if those ways seem "wrong" to me. For example, I've watched a client with a fast respiratory and heart rate tell me they feel "calm" when they are visibly very alert. I simply nod my head and say that's a good descriptor word. "That's remarkable" is another great phrase that does not impose judgment but also doesn't denote agreement. When clients express a feeling that isn't normative, I get curious. Why do they think they are calm when they don't appear to be? I try not to personify animals excessively, but I fall in the camp of personifying them for the benefit of my clients. I might narrate for a rabbit a dialogue in which I project feelings that the rabbit may be having. For example, "Oreo bunny seems to be hiding his face in your lap. Rabbits do that when they feel stressed." Then I might ask what other signs of stress the rabbit is showing (rapid breathing, fast heartbeat, being very still). I might ask if the client ever mimics the rabbit when they are stressed. I might ask how they think we can help calm the rabbit and invite them to identify things that make them feel calm. Sometimes, I go an entirely different direction and lean into the empowerment of the moment. "Oreo seems really scared. Look how he knows you can protect him. I'm so glad you are here to keep my bunny safe today." For some of my clients, their bodies seldom seem safe. The idea of being safe for a soft fluffy bunny can open their minds to new possibilities.

Animals are also great because there is seldom judgment and the interaction is pretty subjective. If you aren't using light pressure or a gentle touch, the animal will likely let you know quickly. They give immediate feedback as to whether the person feels safe or not. Horses are really good at this. Since they are considered a prey animal, they are keen to assess a person's heartbeat and even scent in relation to whether the person feels confident and will help them be safe or is perceived as a threat by the horse. My friend and equine professional, Michael Remole, has said that a horse can tell almost instantly if a client is feeling relaxed or not. He claims that when he uses horses in his psychotherapy sessions, the horse can often tell him things that the client is unable to know themselves at that moment. Whether we use animals or other sensory experiences, helping a client understand their interoceptive sense is pivotal to limbic system rehabilitation.

Suggestions for therapeutic activities that help with **interoception as it modulates feelings and body sensations** taken from the KALMAR app:

- **Feel a variety of textures.** How do the textures feel against your fingers? Your feet? Your arms? Do you like the feeling? Can you describe it? How do you suppose an animal will feel with the same sensations? These questions can help an individual begin to consider how they feel external sensations.

- Find a **variety of sensory experiences** and allow the child to "feel" them. Mirror them, parallel with them. Talk about how you feel and open your curiosity for any reaction they may have that could be the same or different.

- Have the client put their hand on their chest and **count their heartbeat**. How does it compare to a watch that monitors heart rate? Does increasing the heart rate increase the breath? Bringing awareness to internal senses that we feel both internally and externally helps bring awareness to a larger variety of internal sensations. Testing against an app that is objective helps to improve accuracy over time.

- Keep a chart that records **fluid intake** and color of urine. Talk about how thirsty you are each time you drink and how that affects the next urine output based on how much you drink.

- Work with clients so that there is a **"felt-sense" of safety**. As much as possible, allow them control of clothing, food choices, fans, heat packs, etc. Help them get in touch with how sensations feel from their perspective.

CHAPTER 6

• • • •

The Cortex

The cortex is the beginning of our conscious inner thoughts, how we think of objects as a whole, and higher-level processing. It's how we "think" about the sensations we are feeling and how we want to respond to the sensory stimulus we are interpreting from the world around us. It is more evolved in humans than other species, and some say it is what mediates our most "human" characteristics. Looking at drawings or photos of the cortex provides a hint of the many different ways our cortex helps us make sense out of the sensations we feel. There are different separating grooves or sulci that create differently named lobes such as occipital (vision), primary somatosensory (interpreting and responding to sensations), motor (coordinating movement), and parietal (communication). Because it is the most advanced in the brain hierarchy, the frontal lobe, which contains the frontal cortex (personality, morality, and reasoning), will be discussed in the next chapter.

The cortex is responsible for short-term working memory, reasoning, learning, intelligence, organization, executive function, and more. The cortex also gives further understanding and response to many of the sensory sensations that begin their integration in the limbic system. It assists in the coordination of understanding that a horse can be many different sizes, colors, and even representative materials such as plastic toys or elegant bronze statues. Yet all of the items are still called a "horse." While our senses will send conflicting information about weight, size, color, texture, and even smell between different horses, our cortex helps us understand our world better by organizing our perceptions in sensible and patterned formulas. Our cortex labels and organizes experiences in our world and communicates and shares those experiences with others. The cortex influences our creativity, communication, values, sense of time, and even our hopes and dreams.

Functions that are mediated in the cortex (referred to in the KAL-MAR app) that occupational therapists can influence include:

- communication (both verbal and non-verbal)
- sense of time and ability to wait.

Communication (both verbal and non-verbal)

Humans have a deep desire to communicate. There is an adorable video on YouTube called "Listen Linda"[1] where a young boy tries to debate his way into getting a cupcake. At one point, he says, "Linda, LISTEN! You are not LISTENING to me." She then replies, "No. You are not listening to ME." The video is an adorable illustration of the desire to be heard and understood from both people involved. When I'm assessing communication, I look at the client's ability to express needs verbally, answer when their name is called, follow verbal directions, understand conversations, or use appropriate descriptive words.

People who experience adversity often "lose their voice." As I reflect upon the many types of abuse that my clients are overcoming, so many involve silencing them through shame, secrecy, threat, dismissiveness, gaslighting, or non-responsiveness. When they cried, the person who was supposed to comfort or protect them didn't help them. For some of my clients, their voices were literally silenced. I've had some children become selectively mute. Maybe they subconsciously decided their words no longer mattered. When a client stops talking, I see that as a hint that they do not feel safe or valued at that moment. Their brain is so overloaded in that moment that the communication connections have been cut off. Those signals are no longer getting through. Maybe I need to lower my expectations in that moment. Maybe I need to build in cues of felt-safety through rhythm and predictability. Maybe I need to get creative with the way that I communicate with them. I can offer simple one-word choices of yes/no, higher/lower, faster/slower, more/enough. I can help them

---

1   www.youtube.com/watch?v=aFYsJYPye94&ab

use sign language or point to communication augmenters when the mouth simply won't relay the thoughts they have. The further along the arousal continuum tipped towards fear an individual is, the less capacity they have to integrate all of the language processing hubs.

In our cortex, there are many pathways and connections that are working in tandem to synthesize and interpret how a person is standing, their tone of voice, the look in their eye, how they position their hands, the curvature of their mouth, and so many other cues that help us understand the meaning behind their words. University of Texas professor Albert Mehrabian wrote that communication is 55 percent non-verbal, 38 percent vocal, and 7 percent words only. So when an individual struggles with either interpreting or conveying non-verbal communication, it can cause increased confusion as they attempt to interpret what is being communicated as a whole.

Non-verbal communication can also be very tricky and complex for people who have experienced abuse. It's difficult to understand intent when an abuser's body language does not match their words. Some abusers will say they love someone right after they hurt them. As the line in *Wicked* says, "Well, if that's love, it comes at much too high a cost." They may hurt someone and tell them they are fine. So "fine" isn't something they want to feel again. Someone saying "I'm fine" may carry quite the opposite meaning of the actual definition of the words they use. Some of my clients did not have a loving caregiver co-regulating with them and giving them accurate verbal descriptions of their experiences. They gaslit them by telling them their experiences and interpretations were incorrect because the truth would bring a negative consequence or realization of wrongdoing to the caregiver. Or maybe the caregivers had generational trauma and don't have the capacity to co-regulate and find good descriptive adjectives themselves. As Dr. Karyn Purvis used to explain: you cannot take a child to a place of healing that you have not been yourself.

Clients who have experienced confusing or lacking cues of effective communication in their early childhood will need clear examples later in life. Some of my clients become focused on one part of communication and miss the cues they are not tuned into at the moment. They may be so focused on my tone that they miss the words, or they may be taking in so many cues such as my volume, rate of speech, appearance, and other sensory stimuli from the environment that they become overwhelmed and miss parts of the context I'm trying to communicate. For these clients, I need to analyze and scaffold what I'm trying to communicate.

Activities that help with communication often require the therapist to be a keen observer. Is the problem one of state dependence? Will lowering the expectation or stress help? Auditory input can be more confusing and threatening for some clients than visual input. Would communicating visually be better? Can they make simple choices on a visual choice board? Can they tell you a story when you are sitting by their side instead of in front of them? Sometimes having someone next to us is easier than having to consider their body language as we struggle to get our words out. In a tip I learned while working with people with Parkinson's, a simple side-by-side walk can be helpful. Talking is a cadence. It's a give-and-take rhythm. Walking together can increase conversation as the people move in the same cadence and connect physically through the mirrored movements as they connect verbally. With small children, I find lowering the power differential by bending my knees and putting my eye level below theirs can be helpful. Anatomically, when we tilt our head back, it cues our vestibular system to alert us. So allowing the child to have a more flexed pattern sends cues to the child's nervous system that they are safe. Being below them also signals that we do not think we are "above them." We anatomically put them in a calmer position.

Communication is also dependent upon breath support and core stability. For children with low muscle tone, supporting their head so they can see the person they are communicating with can be helpful. If they do not have good breath support to get their words out efficiently, I can work on blowing bubbles or wind instruments. A speech-language pathologist once taught me the trick of bouncing a child seated on a therapy ball up and down while engaging in rhythmic song or words such as a rhyme or counting. She explained how the up-and-down pattern supported the diaphragm and forced air over the vocal cords, making it easier for the child to have the breath support to get the words out. As I mentioned in *The Connected Therapist*, children who talk really fast or really slow might struggle with breath support.

If we have a lot to say and don't have the stability to get it out, we will do it quickly. Higher-pitched words also require less air.

Suggestions for therapeutic activities that help with **communication (both verbal and non-verbal)** taken from the KALMAR app:

- **Oral motor skills** such as blowing-out activities, chewing gum, and speaking with hands close to the throat or mouth for bio-feedback can help rehabilitate communication deficits that are physical in causation.

- Discussion of **communication styles** can be helpful to better understand what an individual is wanting to express.

- **Drumming, singing, and rapping** are activities that help with the cadence, reciprocity, and timing of language.

- Face-focused **collages** can help in identifying facial expressions.

- **Social Stories** (Gray, 2000) can help instill a repertoire of phrases and words to use when an individual has difficulty knowing what to say in social situations.

Sense of time and ability to wait

Fear of the unknown increases our arousal level. Our brain is designed to pay more attention to novel situations and experiences. There is an inherent activation when something is unknown. When the brain cannot rely on predictive patterns, it takes more cortical integration to fully understand what will happen next. Have you ever noticed that your first time driving, biking, or walking a route seems to take longer than once the route becomes more automatic? Our brain defers our sense of time to focus on the unknown task at hand. Dr. Perry's arousal continuum indicates that time, and our ability to think in the future as it relates to time, diminishes as our stress response increases.

With this decreased sense of time as we become more activated, it is really difficult to wait or have patience for delayed gratification.

While on my honeymoon, I overheard a little boy moaning to his parents. His mother said, "Remember, we agreed that we would do that tomorrow." His adorable response was "Yes, but I didn't know today would be sooooo long!" I believe he beautifully expressed how many of us feel as we wait for something we desire. This also makes me think of how pleasant events seem to end too soon but things you don't enjoy seeming to drag on, when, in reality, these events last the same amount of time.

I've had clients who respond well to simply being able to identify that this happens to them, and it is not abnormal. This gives them a feeling of acceptance and helps them decrease their stress response to be better able to access their sense of time. Other strategies I find helpful are letting them know what is coming next. Give them predictability. Let them know how much time it will be and *show* them. Visual timers can be especially helpful because they show how much time has elapsed in a more visual way, accessing the lower-level visual centers when the higher-level sense-of-time center is offline. Some children I work with do well with physically moving stickers or laminated photos to have a tangible way to see the passing of time and task completion. Singing and counting are also ways to help give rhythm and increase predictability of how much time a task will require. Another useful strategy is distraction when waiting is inevitable. Do they *have* to stand in the line? Have you ever had a friend "hold your spot" while you leave the queue to have a walkabout? Can we give children a task to help them pass the time such as watching a short movie clip or engaging them in a game of I Spy? Children who road-tripped in the 1980s could likely give plenty of examples of "ways to pass the time." We played the alphabet game, license plate game, would you rather, and rounds and rounds of bottles on the wall. Helping my clients with waiting and sense of time is often a game of distractions, predictability, and increasing the sense of felt-safety.

Suggestions for therapeutic activities that help with **sense of time and ability to wait** taken from the KALMAR app:

• Drumming and **rhythmic music** stimulates a sense of timing.

- A **wristwatch with a seconds hand** can be a concrete and objective way to witness the passing of time.

- A **fidget** can provide a rhythmic distraction to help with waiting.

- **Social Stories** (Gray, 2000) can ease the anxiety of the unknown when activities involve waiting.

- **Visual schedules/instructions** and visual timers can help with knowing how much time has passed or how much time remains. It can be easier to interpret visual information than auditory information when our arousal levels begin to escalate.

CHAPTER 7

. . . .

The Frontal Cortex

The frontal cortex holds our conscious decisions. It is located within the frontmost outer part of the brain that mediates our thoughtfulness, control, personality, morality, and reasoning. It is how we formulate our opinions and biases based on our past experiences with our surroundings. It has a lot of connections to the other parts of the brain and synthesizes them together in ways unique to each individual. When I worked in a physical rehab setting, a frontal lobe head injury (from a stroke, car accident, or shaken baby) was my most difficult to treat. When someone lost control of one side of their body with a parietal lobe injury, I could give them exercises and a brace and they often regained some independence. If they lost control of the temporal lobe, that was more frustrating because they had difficulty with communication and could be really agitated as they tried to express their thoughts, feelings, and needs. But they usually maintained a level of kindness and I could work with adaptive communication strategies to help them. When a person had a frontal lobe injury, I knew I needed to reach deep within me to find more compassion and hope. Patients with this diagnosis tended to be really emotionally explosive, aggressive, and could be perceived as cruel or manipulative. They lacked functionality of the part of the brain that helped us think of others and want to be agreeable in society.

When I think about this, it helps me to think about the clients I currently treat who have experienced adversity. If they experienced trauma any time before their adult years, chances are pretty good that their frontal cortex is not optimally developed. They may exhibit behaviors, such as impulsiveness, defensiveness, defiance, and avoidance, that I saw in the rehab hospital while working with people who experienced physical injuries. They don't have a visible injury which would have elicited compassion from others. They don't have a history of this compassion from a loving community who sees them through a lens of respect and acceptance. My hope is that this chapter will help you better understand when you see this type of behavior and that the phrase "It's about skill, not will" will return to the forefront of your mind. Because in the forefront of your brain, the frontal cortex is your conscious thought and the lens with which you will view clients who may be labeled manipulative, controlling, and cruel.

Functions that are mediated in the frontal cortex that occupational therapists can influence include:

- impulsivity
- thoughtfulness
- moral reasoning
- delinquent behaviors.

Impulsivity

Impulsivity is developmentally appropriate. Young children truly don't know why taking a toy or cookie is wrong. They lack the life experience, guidance, and mature neural activity in the frontal lobe necessary to have this understanding. I love the TV shows about how kids say the funniest things. They say them because they don't have fully developed frontal cortices. They say them because they are impulsive with their thoughts. They don't "think them through." They believe they can do anything and be anybody. Often the impulsivity of early childhood is very endearing.

When I work with clients who struggle with impulsivity, I need to find the balance between acceptance/nurture and guidance/structure. If I allow a child to simply run wild in my therapy room, it creates chaos within my own nervous system. But if I am too rigid, I run the risk of the child becoming explosive or shutting down in a robotic compliance. As a new sensory-focused therapist, I had heard the phrase "child-led" and found it somewhat confusing. In my own clinical work, I saw so many children who simply ran from place to place, activity to activity within my own space. As I gained experience and leaned into the "therapeutic use of self" model, and began bringing my own regulation to the space, I began to see changes. What this co-regulation looks like is unique because each client is unique. But I've noticed some general patterns. The biggest change has been my letting go of the expectation that I must perform. As a new graduate, I was lucky to have a strong back. I loaded up a heavy suitcase *full* of garage sale crafts and activities to carry from school to school. The idea of not having a fun, goal-directed activity to do every second was terrifying. As a seasoned therapist, I find I need less and less. I'm able to stick with an activity longer myself as my own impulsivity has decreased. I recognized my nervousness and desire to "look like I knew what I was doing" was putting a cloud over my own frontal cortex and making *me* more impulsive.

An example of the difference I'm describing could be a simple task where I use different colored plastic cups and a Lycra hammock swing. The 1996 Marti would have the cups set up in a circle around the swing, ready for the client to be the crashing ball to knock them down. Once knocked down, she would arrange the cups in a particular colorful sequence to make a pattern. There would be music, singing, and a lot of stimulation. I did get results. Kids learned their colors and enjoyed swinging. They did calm a bit simply because I probably exhausted them. I did help them get a little energy out. Plus, I was fun. I was "Fun Marti." I developed a rapport with these children without ever even really thinking about it. I can look back now and see how that rapport and connection through high-energy, silly play was a large part of the therapeutic benefit. I met many of my goals and my payment sources were happy to have me on the team. Looking back, I don't think I was wrong. But I do think I've grown into a better practice model. It honestly makes me excited to see what 2030 Marti will think is best practice, because when I know better, I try to follow Maya Angelou's advice and do better. I'm always learning new things. I hope this book is successful in sharing these new things I learn with other OTs.

The 2023 Marti greets the child at the door and offers a cool beverage or a snack. I watch their body language and meet their energy level. If they are bouncing around as they enter my space, I find a way to match that rhythm. My nearly-50-year-old body doesn't have the stamina of my 20-year-old body. But I can tap my thigh, modify my vocal tone and rate, or change my body posture to influence the non-verbal communication directed at my client. I might still have the plastic cups and the swing. But I'm more confident now to allow the session to unfold a little slower. I'm more OK with the "quiet moments" or the "dead space" between activities. I'm calmer myself and focused to notice the small moments where I can take joy in a little increased eye contact, now aware that we are connecting. When they see the swing and cups, I invite them to play *with* me. I allow them to set them up. If I notice they are setting them up in a random, unstructured way, I look for ways to add structure while still giving them the element of control. Maybe this looks like me having a stack of my own cones that I line up in a certain order or design that slowly provides a visual example of a design option that they may choose to follow as I set mine down. Rather than providing the structure up front, I see how it unfolds in real time. I am modeling less impulsivity by doing things slower with more intentionality. I'm inviting them to co-regulate into this impulse control with me, through connection and felt-safety.

Sometimes I work to help them find an integrative pause. This is sometimes as simple as requesting that the child simply tell me what their next move is going to be. If they want to run around and try out ten different swings, all those steps give me good observations and assessments so I may get curious about what they are seeking. But rather than have them jump off of the bolster swing and run straight into the Lycra swing while yelling across the room, "Next put up the platform swing," I let them know upfront that they may have any swing that they would like. But they should first tell me that they want to move to the Lycra swing and then we give the bolster swing a finalizing transitional swing prior to dismount. Then they can run into the Lycra, and they give me that two-second warning as my assistant is putting up the platform swing. With my most impulsive clients, I find this gives them that element of control and autonomy that they are seeking, while I gently bring in the relationship and the predictability that help them create that integrative pause of understanding and accessing the frontal cortex for their next plan. Thinking back into the sense of time from the cortex, much of impulsivity has to do with that lack of timing and the rhythm that comes with that awareness. So, once again, we can see how these skills and abilities are not independent. The brain does not mediate in isolated functions. It works as a network that must have a strong foundation to integrate the higher structures.

As I gain more experience, I gain more confidence in the still moments. I understand that impulsivity can be experimentation or a fear of doing something wrong. Imagine a client having a paintbrush and they can't create a coherent painting. Rather than draw heavy lines and create tactile boundaries with Wikki Stix or puffy paint, I make it a team project. I allow their marks to be random and haphazard. Then I "Bob Ross" the shared project and paint my happy little clouds and birds on their wild electrical lines and bushes. I *help* my client create beauty *with* me. In the end, they can look at that picture and feel proud of something they created within the context of co-regulation. They build confidence and skill because they stay motivated to complete the task. This doesn't mean I don't use Wikki Stix. I use them when I'm working on visual perception, eye–hand coordination, and even tactile stimulation. But I am also open to allowing the child more autonomy when we are creating art together.

I've had plenty of clients who can't tolerate me adding any of my ideas to their project. If I simply started adding extra lines, that would be offensive to them. They need to do it solely themselves. But maybe I can add structure by inviting them to make marks in rhythm to the platform swing as I'm swinging them. They could put the painting on the floor and make marks as we swing together. I am then less obvious to the client about my co-regulation and input on the activity. If they are having difficulty with stacking cups, maybe I make the cups bigger and fewer to help them be successful with that task. Maybe I hide the cups under heavy weighted blankets or on top of climbing structures for them to retrieve while they get deep proprioceptive input at the same time. As I think through the activity-guiding process, I am reminded how the heart of occupational therapy is function. I hear Tracy Stackhouse's voice in my mind asking, "For the purpose of what?" I am reminded that when I'm working on impulsivity, my purpose is to engage that frontal cortex. To engage the frontal cortex, I need to first calm the brainstem and limbic areas. I need to provide rhythm, predictability, safety, and motivation. Only then can I begin to get curious about ways to practice starting and stopping with intentionality, with the goal of decreasing impulsivity.

Suggestions for therapeutic activities that help with **impulsivity** taken from the KALMAR app:

- **Different types of seating**, such as standing or exercise cushions or balls, provide vestibular and proprioceptive input. This could help meet that need so that an individual isn't jumping around the room seeking the input elsewhere.

- Providing fidgets, weighted blankets, and other **somatosensory supports** can help meet the needs that the individual is trying to find in the environment.

- Providing a **sensory calm area** can facilitate a calming of the brainstem so that the individual is better able to access their frontal cortex to have more mindfulness.

- Proximity to a **regulated and connected caregiver** provides co-regulation and a model for decreased impulsivity.

- Visual schedules, clear expectations, and instructions and demonstration on what is expected can help equip an individual with **practice and understanding** for success.

Thoughtfulness

Thoughtfulness is an interesting concept. When caregivers tell me that their child is not thoughtful, I often rephrase that in my own mind as the caregiver doesn't think that the child is thinking about the things that the caregiver wants them to be thinking about. Usually, it boils down to respect and thinking of the perspective of others. The part of the frontal cortex that deals with perspectives and understanding the viewpoint of another may not be fully engaged or developed for this client.

When I add the lens of trauma, I remind myself and the caregiver that we must have experienced respect in order to be respectful.

We must first have our caregiver think of our needs and our perspectives before we can think of the needs and perspectives of others. If our world view from our early developmental experiences and exposures was that we needed to think of our own needs and perspectives in order to stay safe, it is difficult to put the priority on someone who you may not trust to have your needs and perspectives in mind.

As simple as it sounds, I have found that teaching thoughtfulness requires me to merely be thoughtful. Many of the caregivers I work with struggle with this. It is difficult to give grace upon grace when the child has done something for which society says punishment would be the cure. When our default is to isolate, seclude, and look for payback, these children get very few examples of seeing what thoughtfulness and respect towards another person looks like. They certainly don't see it as an example in their own personal lives. So, in order to change their frontal cortex, we need to change the way we interact with them and how we view the behaviors we see. When we view these behaviors as seeking connection rather than requiring correction, we then can begin the rehab process of teaching a child to be thoughtful and respectful.

In the clinic, this often looks like me talking about my inner thoughts out loud with a very purposeful lens of compassion. When they hit me, I may say, "Ouch, I wonder what made you think hitting me was the best way to move me out of the way. Could you maybe let me know that I am in the path of the ball you were throwing next time? And then when I throw the ball, I will explicitly say I'm going to throw the ball over here because I want to make sure and not hit my friend."

I see every opportunity to praise them and provide suggested language descriptions when they are being thoughtful. I ask thoughtful questions and make statements infused with gratitude. "Oh, thank you for making room for me to sit next to you. I really do enjoy your company." Sometimes, I have opportunities to model how caring for animals can remind us to care for ourselves as well. "Let's give our therapy dog a treat. Do you think she will like this chicken treat? Or this beef treat? Would you like a cold glass of water yourself?" This is yet another reminder of how the frontal cortex hinges on relational security before it can develop.

Another way I encourage thoughtfulness is with a meditative practice. Thoughtful moves or yoga/pilates can help focus the mind on the moment and the movement, helping to quiet external distractors. A sensory space or fidgets can help the child decrease frustrations to better focus and engage the frontal cortex. When I view the skill of thoughtfulness through the lens of connection, experience, and opportunity, I find ways to bring those elements into the therapy room for some pretty great outcomes.

Suggestions for therapeutic activities that help with **thoughtfulness** taken from the KALMAR app:

- Review **state-dependent functioning** to understand if the individual is in a state which allows for cortical processing involving thoughtfulness.

- **Volunteer opportunities** can build empathy and awareness of the needs of others.

- Meditation and other **mindfulness practices** can provide the structure and space/time for accessing the frontal cortex once the brainstem has been calmed.

- Providing a **sensory calm area** so that the individual has access to rhythmic, repetitive, relevant, and rewarding sensory stimuli can help them better access the thinking part of their brain.

- Proximity to a **regulated and connected caregiver** helps cue an individual on expectations. The caregiver can also provide compassionate instruction as needed to help the individual be successful.

Moral reasoning

In order to have moral reasoning, we need to see the perspective of others. As a therapist, I must also recognize that my views and morals are rooted in my own upbringing and community. Moral codes will vary and it's important for me to understand my own biases so that I don't get caught up in defending my own beliefs or trying to rehab things that don't necessarily need to be changed. I remember working in a rehab hospital where a 90-year-old patient with emphysema wanted to figure out a way to hold a cigarette. While I was careful to be sure he wasn't attached to his oxygen tank, you bet I adapted a PVC pipe fitting to help him hold his cigarette. I'm all about quality of life and patient collaboration on goals. While I've never smoked a single cigarette in my life because I have a firm belief in how unhealthy they are, I wasn't about to argue with a 90-year-old man about giving up one of his only remaining pleasures in life. Sometimes, we need to look beyond our own understandings and perspectives as we work to make the lives of our clients better. Sometimes that seems less than ideal based on our own backgrounds. Morals can be similar. They, too, depend on our background as well as our current situations. There are many moral dilemmas about mothers meeting the needs of their babies or people stealing when they are hungry. The more trips I take around the sun, the less black and white the world appears. Often moral-based arguments are controversial because people see the world differently based on their own backgrounds, resources, and abilities to have autonomy.

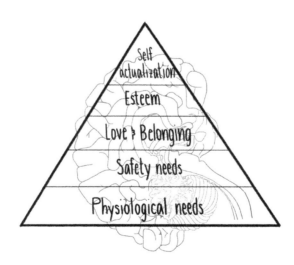

Although we now recognize the cultural biases and limits of this model, Maslow was one of the first to frame our ability to access higher level reasoning and morality as a hierarchy. When our clients are incarcerated or seem to have a "poor moral compass," we must look into their hierarchy of needs. Do they have their physiological needs met? Do they feel safe, loved, and included? Do they believe they have self-worth and the capacity to think creatively and long term? As we look at this hierarchy, we can see the parallels between Dr. Perry's arousal continuum and the brain structure hierarchy that follows that same sequence. Our brainstem is our physiological needs, similar to the Empowering principle from TBRI. Safety, love, and belonging are our TBRI connections found in the limbic system. Then we move forward into the correcting principles of the frontal cortex. Our morals are directly related to how accessible our frontal cortex structures are in that moment.

Different ethics models help us unpack morality. Are we working in the consequentialist theories of utilitarianism (does the greatest good with the least harm), egoism (society benefits when I benefit), or the common good (what is best for the people, especially the most vulnerable). People dedicate entire careers to discussing these theories, because they are incredibly subjective and our view and opinions of them can change based on a variety of circumstances and situations. It is our frontal cortex that helps us decide which theory we will root our decision in. Many of my clients are in the deficiency needs areas of Maslow's hierarchy and therefore often fall into the egoistic category. They can't possibly make moral and ethical decisions based on the needs of others when they don't have their own basic needs met first. With developmental trauma, they may further be lacking the social connections and experience of others caring for them to model how to care for others.

This is helpful to keep in mind as we work with families where the caregiver also has unresolved trauma or where their own physiological, safety, and belonging needs are not being met, as we discussed in the early chapters of this book. There is a lot of wisdom in putting on our own oxygen mask before we can put the mask on those who are dependent upon us.

Social Stories (Gray, 2000) and "what if" scenarios are great ways to engage the frontal cortex. At Simple Sparrow, we use a lot of stories and object lessons with the animals and farmland. We talk about how we have hens who care for chicks they hatch that don't belong to them. We talk about how the llama protects the sheep from predators. We talk about the trust between the farmer and the animals and the seasons of growing. Working in small gardens can foster discussion of how the earth has cycles of seasons and how that impacts communities. Pictorial collages help with imagining moral dilemmas and possible outcomes from various perspectives. Most importantly, we continue to foster relationships that encourage our clients to fully understand how we want the best for them. We trust this process that eventually, when they feel safe and their needs are met, they will begin to consider what is best for others as well.

Suggestions for therapeutic activities that help with **moral reasoning** taken from the KALMAR app:

- Adjust expectations and raise compassion by **understanding the past experiences** and developmental history of the individual. We cannot understand others until we are understood ourselves.

- Volunteer opportunities can promote a **sense of community** and care which can lead to improved moral reasoning.

- Discuss how **animals** care for one another, then relate that to people.

- Be **generous** with the client so they understand what it feels like to have things themselves. This will help disarm the feeling that they need to hoard or steal in order to meet their own needs.

- **Model through example.** Talk about moral situations in your own life and how you are thinking through them.

Delinquent behaviors

Children who experience adversity may have difficulty making friends. They simply were not taught the skills required for social niceties. Encouraging people to like them was less important than getting people to do things for them. They were maybe told that they don't have value, and so they have difficulty seeing their inherent worth. If you engage in delinquent behaviors, it can be an immediately accepting friend group. If our society continues to outcast and ostracize upon the first delinquent act, there is a welcoming community that will quickly trap them in the world of illegal behavior. Once they feel that first burst of acceptance, the alliances are made. It is difficult to get out of trafficked and ganged behavior when you do not know that better communities are a possibility—especially when those "better" communities are the very ones telling you that you don't belong. The sad reality is that while these gangs and groups engaging in illegal acts make the person *feel* valued, the person is actually *treated* as disposable property.

Delinquent behaviors can feel good to our nervous centers. Acts of delinquency cause a spike in excitatory neurotransmitters. For the client who has learned to dissociate to survive, sometimes the thrilling act of the delinquent behavior makes them finally feel alive. Where they have learned to not feel anything to survive the adversity, the delinquency finally brings them up to the level of a normal sensation for someone who does not need to engage in delinquent behaviors. The chemicals that are released in their brain when this happens make it self-reinforcing. For these clients, it can sometimes be successful to introduce new forms of less delinquent adrenaline-seeking behaviors. Riding a motorcycle, skydiving, scuba diving, horseback riding, tattoos, and endurance sports can help release the same chemicals in a more functional manner.

Working in the courts system, many of my clients have involvement with law enforcement and the judicial system. I find it inspiring that this chapter ends with discussion of how my clients often engage in delinquent behavior. As this chapter has hopefully highlighted, much of this behavior is simply because the client lacks the framework to believe other humans will keep them safe and meet their needs. When they were supposed to learn connection, they learned rejection. The treatment for this clinically is to collaborate with trauma-compassionate psychologists, case workers, and caregivers. As the occupational therapist, I work to find ways to build confidence and capacity for co-regulation. I work relationally to decrease shame and build trust. I do everything in my power to echo the words of Dr. Karyn Purvis who worked so hard while she was alive to make sure every child in her program knew they were precious and had inherent worth, regardless of their past. I walk along with the other team members as they help the client reconcile their past while I'm working towards their future. I use my occupational assessment abilities to find occupation and activity that is motivating, interesting, and attainable for my client. I help to empower them so that they can get their needs met within the context of relationship and trust. For so many of the precious people I work with, felt-safety in the context of a trusted relationship *is* the therapy. While it's the simplest therapeutic "activity" to provide, it can be the most difficult to implement if we don't understand the foundational hierarchy of how to rehabilitate people who have experienced trauma and adversity.

Suggestions for therapeutic activities that help with **delinquent behaviors** taken from the KALMAR app:

- Adjust expectations and raise compassion by **understanding the past experiences** and developmental history of the individual. Our client's past environments may have modeled delinquent behaviors that need replacement teaching before they even understand there are other ways to get their needs met.

- **Gardening** is a gentle yet engaging and rewarding hobby that can foster care of the land and community.

- **Teach rather than punish.**

- **Model and parallel leadership opportunities** so they get experience while being supported.

- **Scaffold** situations to promote success. Begin with small tasks and small expectations and then build them up from those experiences.

CHAPTER 8

• • • •

Assessment

This chapter focuses on how I begin to think about my clients through a lens of how their background and current circumstances may influence their current state of functioning. While I sometimes do complete a standardized evaluation when a goal or documentation warrants a specific measure, I tend to use a broader context when I'm formulating my initial assessment strategy.

Paperwork

Assessment for me begins before someone even enters my sensory room. As part of my required paperwork, I ask my prospective clients three questions that I believe to be foundational.

1. Please describe relevant early experiences (birth, adoption, trauma, surgeries, family events, developmental milestones)

For someone who has experienced trauma, it can feel overwhelming to revisit their adversity repeatedly. I want to be sensitive to this. I also want to give my clients a voice in their care. People who experience adversity often feel as though they have "lost their voice." By effectively asking them to tell me the story of the journey that brought them to me as the first interaction I have with them, I am letting them know that they will have a voice with me. So often, there is no checkbox for the situations my clients experience. Their family history is complicated and complex. Standardized forms can evoke shame, frustration, and even confusion for many of my clients who experienced early childhood trauma.

A narrative opportunity can give me such insight into where my client is in their trauma-awareness journey. I've had people say very little in this area only to discover their early experiences are actually very complex and tragic. Sometimes this gives me insight into their dissociation from reality, or simply their fatigue in having to constantly explain themselves. I might learn that the caregiver doesn't understand how traumatic an early adoption can be. They may not understand that even though the child was adopted at two days old, their entire in utero experience was filled with adversity. They don't understand how the brain structures that mediate our sense of safety and well-being were influenced by that in utero experience. Or maybe they write so little because the constant retelling is exhausting for them.

I've had other clients fill pages with specific details. This, too, gives me insight into how they are approaching their therapeutic journey. When I see pages of detail, I can be curious about whether that person needs validation that things are so very difficult or there is a complexity that they hope I can untangle. I can gain insight for just how complex the trauma really is for this family. For some, it simply provides a framework for them to consider for themselves how birth, adoption, trauma, surgeries, family events, and developmental milestones might influence the current function for the client that warrants therapy. If nothing else is accomplished, I hope it sets the foundation for my clients that I value their input and I plan to include them in the therapeutic process.

2. Please tell me what has or hasn't worked in the past in regard to previous therapies (OT, physical therapy, speech therapy, play therapy, counseling, animal-assisted therapy, auditory programs, special treatment places/protocols)

For many of my clients, I'm often not their first stop. They have tried other therapies, models, treatments, and programs. This question gives me a good starting point and helps me not waste their time and resources exploring things that haven't been successful. Answers to this question can evoke a curiosity in me of their capacity to follow through if I see they have tried many things. It can show me their outlook on various approaches if they expand on whether or not it worked. This question helps to guide me in regard to what places this family has already visited on their roadmap to treatment. It gives me some common language and understanding of various approaches and helps me identify patterns in their therapeutic journey.

3. Please give me at least three goals for our time together. Why are you wanting OT services? What would you like for your child to accomplish?

Insurance companies have so many restrictions around this, and many continuing education courses focus on goal writing. I'm surprised that it doesn't seem more common to simply ask the caregiver why they have come to therapy. It seems so obvious. So often, however, it is left to the professional to decide. Sometimes, it's left to the third-party payer to decide. In a space where narrative, having a voice, and feeling a sense of control is so important, I want to empower my clients with this question. Yet I am surprised by how many of my clients simply say, "Tell me what to do." When overwhelmed, they may say, "Evaluation" or "Regulation." It is almost always something very general. This unspecified generalization tells me they are so deep in the trauma expression that they don't even know what goals are possible.

Other times, I read very specific goals that I can immediately tell are evidence of incredibly high expectations being put on the client from the well-intended caregiver. This question can lead me to an understanding of the way a caregiver disciplines when I read words like "obey," "respect," "listen," or "achieve." This also helps me frame how I am going to interact with the caregiver to ally with them in hopes of helping them see if there is a need to change some of the narrative they have about their child's motives and capabilities. This question helps me prioritize where to begin our sessions. When the goals are to listen, calm down, etc., I know we will be starting with goals of co-regulation for both the child and the caregiver.

Initial interaction

Once I have the requested paperwork, I start going through my mental Rolodex of things I have learned, courses I have taken, methods I have studied, and words of people I admire. While I am capable of standardized testing and do sometimes find it useful, much of my assessment is done through observation and dialogue with the caregiver and the child at a level that is respectful and appropriate. I often think of my first interaction with my clients as a "thinking or pondering out loud session." I literally say a lot of phrases out loud in front of the clients, such as:

I wonder if:

- I wonder if they feel comfortable.

- I wonder if they are showing me what they are capable of.

- I wonder if they are being silly because this task is too hard.

- I wonder if they do better with this task if they have their glasses or medication.

- I wonder if the caregiver sees this action at home.

- I wonder if this behavior is expressed at school.

- I wonder if changing a position or providing a therapeutic assist will make them successful.

- I wonder if anyone has ever asked you about your preference with this.

- I wonder how you feel if I say you look really guarded in this position.

Have you ever noticed/do you notice:

- Have you ever noticed if you get dizzy in the car?

- Have you ever noticed that noises bother you?

- Have you ever noticed that you seem to prefer your right arm to your left? I wonder if your right arm is stronger.

- Do you notice how your past provided you with really good survival strategies you may not need anymore?

- Do you notice how you eat your food quickly? Do you enjoy the food you eat? Do you think about how it feels or tastes in your mouth?

- Do you notice how your shoulders appear to be rounded forward in that chair as opposed to more straight across on the therapy ball?

What happens when/if:

- What happens when we uncross your legs? Add a weighted lap pad? Turn your chair around?

- What happens if I give you a little less verbal instruction paired with more processing time?

- What happens when I add or subtract things from your environment, like bringing in a therapy animal or trusted friend or removing some visual clutter?

- What happens when I change your body position as you swing?

Much of my "thinking out loud" is to put the client at ease. I'm not looking for ways to judge or shame them. I'm simply looking at things with an objective and physical lens. It allows them to know why I'm asking them to do weird body positions. For many people who experience trauma, things were done to their bodies where they felt out of control. People who hurt them would interact with them physically in ways that were not respectful or pleasant. It can feel very vulnerable to have a stranger ask you to move in certain ways or complete unknown or puzzling tasks without an understanding of the reason behind the movements and activities.

Thinking out loud also opens a dialogue where they can help guide me. It helps them feel that they are a part of their treatment plan and care. When I think out loud, they can hear in my voice how wonderful, valuable, and precious I think they are. I can demonstrate verbally for them how I believe they are doing their best and their body is simply functioning in a way that is keeping them safe. Instead of shaming them for talking so loudly all the time, I can "wonder if you can hear the volume of your voice compared to mine (or your dad's or this chicken's)." I add the chicken example because, of course, a chicken will be loud. For a child who needs to learn in the extremes before they can regulate themselves to the middle of the volume range, a chicken squawk or other non-judgmental and interesting noise such as a truck horn can be a great non-shaming comparison. So many of my clients are already comparing themselves to other humans and are reactive to their deficits in that comparison.

When I "think out loud," I can wonder if they don't eat broccoli because it scatters erratically in the mouth and is difficult to orally motor plan. The client or caregiver then has the opportunity to wonder themselves if they never considered that. Or they have the opportunity to correct me and say it's actually because they dislike the color green and steak, cauliflower, carrots, and chicken wings are complex foods that they actually enjoy.

Match expectations

When I first began my "trauma-informed" journey, I remember Dr. Perry teaching us to raise our compassion and empathy while better matching our expectations to the child's raw ability. We also need to consider their motivations and perceptions *in each moment*. Before studying Dr. Perry's model of state-dependent functioning, I didn't fully consider that ability was fluid. It is, as the model articulates, state dependent. Much of the standardized testing I learned in OT school had the evaluator present a task and see how the child performed. They either completed it successfully or they didn't. There wasn't an area to score for how the child's morning routine was interrupted or if they were nervous about a new place or if the decor in my office reminded them of something unpleasant or pleasing. Learning about state-dependent functioning helped open my clinical reasoning skills to consider that a child may perform a task differently in any given moment. It helped me make goals that considered other factors besides testable abilities.

Most four-year-olds are physically able to put their shoes on independently and get in the car within a five-minute period. It seems like a reasonable expectation and goal. When the dog just tore through the house with the end of a toilet paper roll and the baby is crying, this toddler may still be expected to do this sequence independently as the parent is screaming "Bad dog!" while clutching the bouncing baby under their arm and chasing a stream of white through the kitchen. While the expectation was reasonable in the quiet moment prior, the expectation obviously needs to be lowered with the distraction and humor of the chaos surrounding the kitchen island. What if the parent is violent towards the dog? What if the baby needs to be set down unattended as the dog is creating a parent obstacle course game of chase? Does it change the perceived level of expectation if we know the early adversity of the child? Maybe they were often left in charge of their baby siblings. Maybe there was a dog that bit them in the past and this dog seems out of control. Maybe there was a lot of yelling and chasing in their past that was followed by abuse. When we begin to add in outside factors that may be drawing the toddler's attention away from the task and into their own felt-safety in the moment, we can begin to see how their ability to successfully complete the expectation is dependent on how their past intertwines with the current moment. While this is a pretty extreme example, it can lead us to consider the child who is able to complete the standardized testing adequately in my little broom-closet OT room but falls apart in the classroom. It can lead us to consider the teenager who fails a test of content they know after a conflict on social media. It can help us set the stage for actual success in the future by considering more underlying factors.

A teenager can clean their room when their friend is coming over. But when they have a bullying experience at school, or they have a looming test they don't feel confident about, or the individual they have a crush on posts about a romantic interest on social media, they lose that capacity. Asking them to clean their room while their brain is focused on those events will likely result in an unmet expectation. They may need more support such as a buddy to co-regulate with them, motivation of something powerful enough to refocus their mind, or more simple-step direction such as "just put your dirty laundry in this hamper."

I see this represented in my clinic by the parent who claims that the child is able to function well at school but falls apart when they get home. Or the spouse is very high-achieving at work but then isn't very engaged at home. The perception is these individuals seem to give their best to others and fall apart around the ones they believe won't abandon them. The reality is they may simply not have anything left to give. The internal motivation to pay their bills or succeed at school may keep them in a state of high robotic compliance between the hours of 8 and 5. But they simply don't have anything left to give the rest of the day as they become fatigued.

This is a really important concept to grasp as we raise empathy and compassion and match our expectations to appropriate levels. When we view the situation or event as personal or "against us," we tend to be judgmental and harsh. But when we realize that our brains simply can't function on high demand all the time, we can have some compassion and lower our expectations. We can build scaffolding and support while better prioritizing the absolute goals of the situation.

If my four-year-old isn't able to put their shoes on in a chaotic moment, maybe they will put their shoes on in the car when things have settled down. I had a friend during my early child-raising years who simply stored all the children's shoes in the back of her van to keep life simple. Other solutions include simplifying the shoes to slides or non-lace options, buying fewer styles of shoes and buying multiples of the same shoes that are used the most so it's easier to find the match, cutting a sticker in half and putting it in the heels so they can better line up which foot is which, or attempting to put the shoes on before the chaos of packing up the car begins. Allow more time. Allow more flexibility. Allow more guidance. Allow more grace for the expectation.

If my teen isn't able to clean on demand, maybe I can set a timer for a reasonable amount of time that they can spare. Maybe I can create a system of bins that are easier to maintain. Maybe I join alongside them and help them so they don't feel overwhelmed. I look for connection while I'm teaching them organizational and cleaning techniques that will carry them into adulthood. Maybe I learn to simply care less. My children are currently 13 and 16. For years, I have had a little sign in their bathroom (which doubles as our guest bathroom) that says, "My children are graciously sharing their bathroom with you. It was clean yesterday. Sorry you missed it. If you have cleanliness concerns, please utilize the cleaning wipes under the sink." Most of my guests see the sign as humorous. Seldom do the wipes get utilized. I remember my own mother once requiring "a path that a fireman could access your bed through this pile of belongings." That seems like a realistic expectation with a loving motivation. I've used that same line with my own children.

On days when work is stressful, I adjust the budget to account for pre-cooked meals, because cooking is not relaxing to me but providing nutritious food for my family is. My husband lovingly teases me as I justify our finances using "Marti Math," meaning I work numbers illogically to land in my favor. But I simply consider it refinancing. If I'm stressed at work, I'm probably not able to go to Target. So, that budgeted $100 Target trip (no matter if you went in for one thing or 40) can be re-shuffled to the food budget. If I'm too stressed to feed my family, I probably don't need that adorable Target seasonal decor I won't get around to putting out anyway. If you were to visit my home as I'm writing this book, you might find that I have dishes in the sink, and I've gained a few pounds as I'm sitting more and scrubbing my floor less. You might also find me sitting in my pajamas under the summer glow of the winter Christmas tree lights. I'm not prioritizing cleaning or decorating with an extra project on my plate. But I'm also not missing any school performances or dinners out with friends. I have my priorities and I try to help my clients find theirs.

These changes in expectation are a reflection of the awareness that no one can maintain perfection all the time. We simply aren't meant to. As our brains constantly work to maintain balance, so must we. I hope you can find the grace not only for those you interact with but also for yourself as you work to match the expectations to the current capacities of yourself and of the individuals you work with.

When an individual is in the alert state of functioning, they may demonstrate avoidance strategies in an attempt to make sense of their experience. They may say, "I don't know" in response to a question. They may claim they don't know *how* to clean their room or put on their shoes, even though they have demonstrated this ability to you countless times in the past. When we start to notice these patterns and cues, we can better interact with the individual by increasing their support. We might decrease our language and increase our non-verbal signs of safety. We might offer to meet their basic needs by inviting them to have a cup of tea or a snack of fruit or, more enticing...cookies, gasp! Cookies are not "rewards for bad behavior" when offered as a regulatory strategy. Once their state of functioning begins to soften through that external support (co-regulation), then we can begin to use very simple language to indicate that we will continue to support them on their task. We might offer to sit in the room with them so they can ask us questions on where things should be placed if they are cleaning, or hand them their shoes if finding them was simply too difficult at that moment.

Often, people new to this concept challenge that it is too permissive. I have found in my practice that most people desire independence. Indeed, occupational therapists have devoted our entire careers to the concept of helping people be independent with tasks of daily living. I once saw a delightful video clip of a young girl, maybe three years old, instructing her presumed father to "just drive" while she worked diligently to buckle her own seatbelt, repeatedly saying, "I do it myself...you take care of yourself." Developmentally, "I do it myself" is normal and frequent. Many of us don't even outgrow it, bearing in mind how much difficulty we have accepting help as adults. This brings us back to the idea that children who *know* what to do and are *able* to do it in *that moment* (that survival-depending moment of state of function) do well.

I am encouraged that OT students are beginning to ignite an interest in trauma assessments and treatment. I look forward to the day when there are well-known standardized evaluations and evidence-based protocols for treatment of people who have experienced trauma and adversity. The reality is that "trauma" is as diverse as the people who experience it. If our "norms" are calculated by normative studies, it is impossible to have a standardized outcome for such a norm-diverse population. As of this writing, I simply find the approach in this chapter to be a good fit for my individual practice. As a founding board member of A-TROT (Alliance of Trauma Responsive OT Practitioners), it is my desire to work with other OTs to bring both awareness and clarity to this practice of being "trauma informed."

CHAPTER 9
• • • •

Working in Different Environments

The activities we choose are directly dependent upon the location where they will be implemented. Many public institutions don't allow gum for oral motor regulation. In a school, the gum tends to end up under the desk and on the carpet. If we are fortunate, we can make accommodations by only chewing in the OT room, with the assurance of proper final disposal, or during specific monitored times. In a locked facility, gum can be used to "gum up" the locks and be a security concern. Because of this, it is necessary to be aware of how the therapeutic activity will be used and the cooperation and input from the caregivers and staff who may be affected by the implementation. For this reason, the KALMAR app has the option to choose between locations such as school, home, and farm when generating activity suggestions.

In addition to location, we must consider the uniqueness of each individual. It's important to think through potential side effects or past associations. I've had several clients whose fear response increases based on physical attributes of a person who reminds them of an abuser. Some clients feel restrained by a weighted blanket when they aren't introduced to it with full autonomy and ability to control its use and removal. Since smell is so closely associated with PTSD and memories, certain perfumes, substances like alcohol and marijuana, and cleaning products can transport an individual back to times when their bodies did not experience felt-safety. It is important to consider cultural differences as well. Certain foods, hand gestures, clothing, and even eye contact can be perceived differently than intended. I have found that the best way to discover possible unintended consequences is to be very curious and ask questions. I read the body language of my client and look for things in the environment that seem to make them more or less comfortable. If they are pulling towards midline, pacing back and forth, turning their back to me, or even coughing, I become curious about whether something is overwhelming for them at that moment. I then do an environmental "safety check" where I try to see the sensory surroundings from their perspective as best I can.

Safety is another consideration based on setting. If I am in a larger group setting, I need to be mindful of how much supervision the activity I recommend requires. Swim noodles in a group of two people looks very different from swim noodles in a group of 20 people. Can the items I am suggesting be used as a weapon? When I work with incarcerated youth, I need to be mindful of things that could be used as a rope or sharp object. Writing utensils need to be soft, like crayons and pastels. Paints need to be non-toxic. Balls for throwing need to be squishy and not too firm to prevent injury. I'm constantly asking myself if the activity could hurt the client, myself, or others. When there is a high likelihood of destruction, I also ask myself if I'm OK for that object to be damaged. Is it disposable? When I can, I try to provide enough trust and rapport where I can feel more confident with allowing "riskier" objects. But I do so with understanding that things may get a little crazy and I have well-designed back-up plans for quick cessation of the activity if it gets hazardous.

In my work with the juvenile justice systems and family courts, I'm encouraged by a trend of more family support and caregiver compassion. Where judicial and legal systems used to be focused on punishment, they are slowly shifting to a more rehab-focused model. One of the most inspiring scenarios I have the privilege of being a part of is seeing a juvenile correctional dorm adopt the TBRI model as a study. I was brought in to assist with creating an environment that would stimulate the senses in purposeful ways. Originally, there were harsh, cold walls in dirty gray tones. They switched the paints to warm nature and blue tones and added murals for interest. They took a risk and put carpet and rugs in some areas where children used to utilize creative means to damage the flooring. What they are finding is that the children feel trusted and respected. The staff assumed that providing basic comforts would lead to those items being destroyed, but the children actually began taking care of those upgraded and comforting items. So many "institutions" lack interest and stimulation. The stimulation they did have was often negative. Without pictures on the walls, the noise echoed, and a small outburst was quickly perceived as violent and would then escalate to actually become more violent. With bare walls and staff touch rules in place, children lacked the tactile stimulation that their developing sensory systems craved. Without this external tactile stimulation, they became fecal artists and engaged in self-harm to "feel" things. While the staff had to be careful that objects could not be used as weapons, they made some very positive changes. Children were given choices of scented soaps and hand sanitizers. They were offered mints and flavored waters. Sturdy canvases were hung on the wall to dampen noises and wireless speakers provided pleasant ambient sounds.

I had several staffings where we discussed simple developmentally appropriate ways to adjust the sensory stimulation for children serving longer sentences. We discussed how a loud slamming cell noise would be scary for any ten-year-old. We talked about reading bedtime stories, allowing a small soft "lovie" blanket, and providing other age-appropriate ways to connect and meet tactile needs. We added felt to the metal bars so that they did not sound so alarming when they shut. We adjusted the lighting in the hallway to be a softer night light instead of blaring bright light. Instead of sounding an alarm when it was time to go to bed, they played a soft chime over a wireless speaker. An interesting observation I made was how many children converted to the Muslim religion so that they could have a prayer rug in their cell. Often, that was used not only for prayer, but also as a silky sensory sheet and a way to bring some color to their room. I noticed children who rubbed toothpaste or bodily substances on the plastic guards that covered the lights to decrease the glare before warmer colored bulbs were used. When the environment is not pleasing to our senses, we have an innate desire to make things more pleasing. We want our homes to be an expression of ourselves and our preferences. Allowing children the trust and respect to make these small changes had lasting carry-over to the trust and respect they showed to others.

Another positive program I've seen in places where there are rules against touch is to add animals that can be petted and cuddled.

Long-term care facilities that allow therapy animals tend to have positive outcomes in regard to social and tactile development. One of my favorite animal experiences was when we took chicks to a senior assisted-living facility. The residents loved feeling their soft feathers and tiny little feet. They were engaged and reminiscent of days past when they lived in rural farm areas and raised their own chickens. The sweet sound of the peeping mixed with the other tactile sensations encouraged the residents to engage the memory portions of their brain as well as social connectedness as they shared in a communal sensory experience.

I have heard some great sensory suggestions after consulting with agencies that support foster families. One of my favorites, from Dr. Karyn Purvis, is to have pre-made break-and-bake cookies on hand so the child is greeted immediately with warm cookies and a sweet aroma upon arrival at a new placement home. Providing a tour and letting them know where they will sleep, toilet, and have a place for just them to relax is important. Children in the foster system often come with food insecurities and toileting troubles. Much of this is due to the lack of routine, structure, and predictability in their day-to-day lives. I instruct caregivers to never lock up food and to have healthy foods in easy-to-consume individual portions available. If the child tends to hide food, offer less rodent-attracting options such as cereal bars that are individually wrapped and easily consumed in one sitting. Individually wrapped sugar-free mints are also a good option because they are a natural bug deterrent and provide a nice sensory "boost" in a small package that doesn't leave a decaying peel. They are inexpensive and even do well when going through the wash in forgotten pant pockets.

Places with high turnover can benefit from cute labels on things to aid a child in orienting to their surroundings. Stickers (cut out of vinyl on a special cutting machine used for crafts) on the toilet, closet, pantry, and linen doors can be a cute way to help a child have independence in unfamiliar environments. When giving tours and orienting new children, it is best to keep verbiage positive. Instead of saying, "This is the food reserved for dinners. Don't eat things on this shelf," you could say, "This shelf has unlimited snack-sized things you are welcome to eat in the kitchen or on the porch. Please put wrappers in the bin labeled 'trash' when you are done." I have seen places where each child is given a plastic bin labeled with their name or a character that is meaningful to them. Offering a child who is often uprooted a place to store things as their very own space can send a powerful message of security. Whereas locking a child out of things like a pantry, closet, or even room can send a message of distrust and heighten curiosity and a desire to gain access, giving them the key to their own lock box (that maybe are kept in a safe place where the adult also has access, but not other residents) can give them a sense of control and power that they lack and may be seeking in other ways.

When providing adaptive or sensory equipment in schools and other places with high numbers of people, I find a variety of sensory supports such as weighted blankets, fidgets, seating options, scented items, and adaptive supplies like pencil grips, built-up handles, and spring-loaded scissors can be helpful. When something new is first introduced, there is often a curiosity and desire to explore in many of the children. However, as the novelty wears off, the children seldom choose adaptive supplies unless they specifically need them. Often, I bring two of the items I want my client to use. One for them and one for a friend. This helps eliminate jealousy or making my client feel "different."

When I go into any space, I try to imagine what my clients and others in the space are experiencing. I ask myself to explore sensations. What do I see? I wonder if things are too bright or too dimly lit and how the colors and backgrounds evoke feelings of safety or threat to my nervous system. What do I smell? I wonder if there are smells that would be offensive or smells that could be intentionally and strategically used to evoke pleasant sensations for the client. I look at where the smell is located and if I can make it stronger or weaker if I want to. I am curious who gets to choose the smells. What do I feel? I wonder if children can go barefoot or if the staff members are allowed to give them safe touch and proprioceptive hugs. If they are not allowed, I look for other opportunities to get these needs met. What do I hear? I listen for background noises, ambient noises, noises that could be startling. I ask if my clients are able to control the noises they hear with music options, white-noise machines, or noise-canceling headphones. What is the food and water situation? I wonder if food and water are readily available and inviting, as a signal of care. I wonder what supports are in place and if the staff are considering sensory stimulation as part of the treatment plan. I then wonder many of the same things as I consider the working environment for the support staff who are working with the children I'm serving. Because I've learned that the best way to provide sensory support to my clients is to first provide it to the caregivers. It helps to "feel" the difference themselves if I want to encourage buy-in and stamina as I ask them to try new things.

CHAPTER 10

Community and Caregiver Considerations for Treatment Planning

Humans, including caregivers, match others around them, especially when they are stressed. When a child grows up in a stressful environment, their brain changes to be very adept at finding non-verbal cues of threat. They become hypervigilant. When they move to that hypervigilance, they lose the capacity to really think about the things they are experiencing and often will presume a situation is more dangerous than it actually is. They miss cues of safety because their brain is not practiced in finding cues of safety.

Caregivers who live in these stressful situations with children who themselves do not feel safe often report feeling unsafe as well. These feelings are substantiated with real acts of violence that then bias the caregiver's brain to also be over-vigilant. This over-vigilance then carries over to circumstances and relationships outside the home. Caregivers become disconnected from the community. They don't have a support network that can help them practice a calm state of arousal. They may interpret benign acts as aggression or assume no one wants to interact with them. As a community, we must consider what ways we can help support these caregivers and their children. Rather than isolate and shame when something happens outside of the social norm, we can think, "Why did this happen?" If we are punishment and isolation focused, the children do not have the opportunity to practice the preferred social expectations and the caregivers lose the momentum and motivation to keep going. The alarmingly high number of disrupted foster placements prior to aging out of the system is evidence that many children lack the sustained practice that is needed to build neural connections of inclusion, belonging, safety, and unconditional love and acceptance. When we understand the why behind the behaviors, the focus moves from punishment to prevention. We can come alongside the caregiver and help them borrow our state of calm (co-regulate) to help move them back to a state of calm with us. When we support the caregivers, we are supporting the children in their care.

Because of their overwhelm, I'm unable to provide intense home programs and parent education in the beginning of our treatment relationship. I find that too many of the parents I work with feel abandoned themselves. They feel unseen, unheard, uninspired, unconfident, and exhausted. I must help the parents feel seen and help them move out of their alert and terror states. I must help them find community. I must help them feel seen, heard, and validated. Being seen is one of the best ways to increase felt-safety. Robyn Gobbel created an online forum for caregivers who have children who require extra compassion and care called The Club.[1] As I've seen this community grow, I'm encouraged by how just knowing there is someone else who understands how they feel can be so empowering and hopeful. For many of my clients, this is the foundation of my work with them. My hope is that the work of my trauma-compassionate colleagues alongside me will bring awareness to better community support and respite for these families who are fighting so hard to help children who have been hurt learn to not hurt others.

When we experience adversity, we look around and see how others will react. When a fire alarm goes off, we look to the leader in the room. But sometimes our leaders aren't equipped to handle the emergency themselves. Some leaders are trying to make those emergency decisions without a practiced neural pattern to follow. Our children from adversity can assume the role of the unpracticed leader. They may have been left alone or with younger siblings to care for and acquired survival skills that are effective at survival but inhibit connection. They have strong neural learning that they themselves are the only

---

1   https://robyngobbel.com/theclub

individual capable of keeping themselves safe. They might be able to get themselves out of the burning room, but they might use other less familiar humans in the room as tools, because no one ever demonstrated to them how to lead. No one showed them there were other routes to safety and meeting their needs.

I recently had a discussion about a person taking three pieces of pizza because they were afraid it would run out (leaving less for themselves) and a person who took one piece of pizza because they were afraid it would run out (leaving less for others). So much of our survival and protective patterns depend on the people around us and our assumptions based on our past memories of how they will keep us safe and care for our needs. So much of a person's felt-safety and ability to think beyond the moment depends on their perceptions of the people who are in charge. When the people in charge appear stressed, the children in their care lose trust.

Thus, the cycle of self-preservation for both child and caregiver continues. Therefore, when I am thinking through my assessments within my clinic space, caregiver arousal state and community support capacity are important considerations. Therapist Nikki Noteboom once said to me, "Heal the mother. Heal the child." I've taken that advice to heart and do my best to bring that into my own clinic space. Sometimes, that looks like offering compassion and connection through a cup of coffee or cold bottle of water. Sometimes it is taking five minutes while the child is otherwise engaged and asking how the week is going or asking if they have any questions. It is something I consider when I begin to think about home programs or homework.

CHAPTER 11

Practical Equipment Suggestions

After the birth of my daughter, I opened the front room of my own home as a certified outpatient clinic in Texas. I first opened the space as a way to work from home while financially writing off the sensory equipment I needed for my own child. Then I realized how powerful home intervention can be. Because of this, I strive to keep equipment easy to install and inexpensive. I want the clients I treat to participate in therapy sessions and be empowered to create their own "sensory room" where my treatment suggestions can be practiced and carried out with more repetition than one or two times a week in my clinic space. My newest sensory space is in a farmhouse. We converted the front dining area into a therapy room by simply laying down a wrestling mat, blocking the hallway with shelves, and putting a few eye hooks in the studs of the walls and ceiling. Most of my "equipment" is made from inexpensive items purchased from the local hardware store or online, or I find it in my Buy Nothing group (a local Facebook group where neighbors can request and gift items for free that they no longer need). In this chapter, I will give suggestions on how I create some of my favorite therapeutic "tools" on a limited budget.

Vestibular and proprioceptive sensory input are cornerstones to my therapeutic interventions. When I first started working at the care farm, I installed an inexpensive round net swing from Amazon. com on the ceiling rafters in the barn. My clients would swing with the chickens and goats, and it was a lovely way to match the energy of the farmyard. I still use that inexpensive swing today. I also use a swing I created out of an IKEA tabletop. Since the tabletop I am using is square, I add a swim noodle to the outer edges to protect myself and anyone else in the room as those corners are flying around. To suspend the swing, I drill holes in each of the four corners of the table, place a vinyl or other water-resistant material over the table, and cut holes in it that line up with the ones I just drilled. I then put a washer above and below the holes for stability. I next thread 3–4 feet of rope through the holes and washers and make a large knot on the bottom of the swing. I'm not fancy with my knots. I typically just tie it many times until the knot is large enough that it feels secure. Most times, the swing is in my hands and if the knot did pull through, the child would be fine as they land either in my lap or on top of a 3-inch foam mat from an 8-inch height. Once I have the knots secured, I make square knots to tie them all together to a sturdy carabiner that has a weight capacity of at least 300 pounds. To reinforce this top connection and keep the ropes from swinging around, I use duct tape to wrap around the base of the carabiner that is securing the ropes. Since I typically have tools, rope, and duct tape on hand, if I can find a donated table top, this swing costs me less than $25 and about an hour of my time.

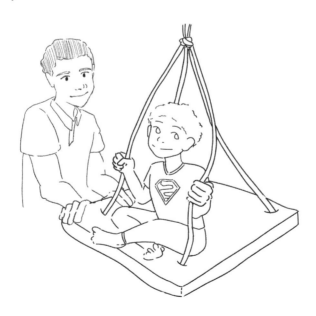

The **platform/tabletop swing** is great for spinning and times when I want the child to criss-cross applesauce (cross legs as in the illustration) or be on their belly with more support. But sometimes I prefer a **bolster swing**. Bolster swings are often viewed as a more rehab-coded product and are not as available commercially. But I wanted to keep my cost lower than what is offered in the therapy catalogs. When my oldest was little, I discovered that she loved the garden section of a large home improvement store. To regulate both of our nervous systems, I often found myself walking the aisles of the home improvement stores with a baby strapped to my body in a sling. Being a clever OT who loves to adapt things on a budget, I would simply wander around wondering, "How could I use this with my patients?" On one such stroll, I encountered cardboard tubes that are intended to hold concrete in place while it dries for making large poles that hold large lights, like you see in parking lots. The interesting thing about these cardboard tubes is they come in sizes that are only a few inches different in circumference. They do this for a bigger shipping capacity, because these poles don't need to be exact sizes. Yet these cardboard tubes are incredibly sturdy to hold the wet concrete in place as it dries and hardens. I discovered that if I nest two of them together and duct tape some pipe insulation tube or a swim noodle on the end, it functions just as well as the expensive bolster swings I see in the rehab catalogs. Just as I do with the tabletops, I drill holes through the nested tubes, reinforce them with washers, and attach ropes. I also add an additional loop around the tube so that the force isn't solely on the drilled holes. To keep the children from sliding around, I add a yoga mat with duct tape as well. Each of these tubes costs $10–$20. I've never had one break in nearly 20 years while children of all sizes ride their rockets to the moon and horses across the country. With a bolster like this one, I can work on flexion as they hold on to the "rocket ship" or hang from the "tree branch" like a sloth. If I need to add some rhythmic proprioceptive input, I bounce the bolster against my body or a large therapy ball. A favorite in my therapy room is to stack plastic cups and ram them down with the bolster. This is also a great tool for relationship work. I can have two people sitting on either end, either facing away from or towards each other depending on the level of comfort and connection. This is an excellent way to respectfully get two people on the same beat/rhythm to help them co-regulate as they share a felt sensory experience.

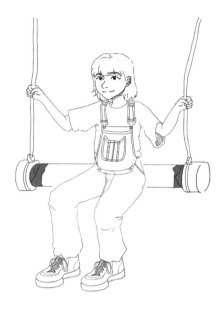

I can usually find heavy-duty swivel swing hangers online for around $15–20 that drill directly into the studs in my ceiling. Since most of my swings hang rather low and are used with supervision, I find the biggest risk is the hardware falling and hitting a child on the head if the hook comes out of the ceiling support stud. Because of this, I secure another eye bolt to the next stud over where I can tie a piece of rope between that eye bolt and the swivel swing. This way, if the swing breaks loose, it will catch on the rope and remain in the air attached to the other stud.

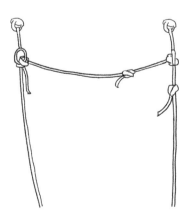

The swing I most often use is my **Lycra nest swing**. I use three yards of Lycra, folded in half and sewn along the edges and then folded at the ends and sewn to make a channel for the rope. The rope is threaded through the channel, tied into individual circles on each end, and attached to the ceiling rope with a carabiner. If I want the swing to be more open, I attach it to two hanging ropes. If I desire a more teardrop function, I clip the two ends together to make a single point of attachment. This swing is a favorite for promoting a calming flexion pattern while I provide either rhythmic or chaotic movement to the vestibular system. If I am looking to match high energy or increase the arousal, I might start with chaotic/non-rhythmic swinging. To bring the client back to calm, I might move more rhythmically and adjust the beat/timing/quickness to suit the therapeutic goal.

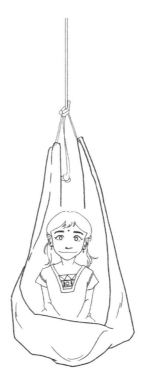

For all of my suspension equipment, I find it helpful to have an adjustable carabiner and rope that does not fray. This makes switching out swings quick and easy.

I've been known to claim old **swing-set slides** from my local Buy Nothing group on occasion and simply place them on the stairs. When I don't have access to them for free, I fold a piece of cardboard in half and place it on my existing stairs. It makes a great recycled slide, especially for rainy-day fun. I place a pillow at the base of the stairs and the kids have a blast. If I feel extra cautious, I'll add a bicycle helmet to the fun. While I don't fully recommend it for liability reasons, I'd be remiss if I didn't write about my most epic slide event with my own children. I covered a mattress with satin sheets and sent my babies sailing down the stairs. Thankfully, everyone lived. My now-teenagers still talk about that day nearly a decade later.

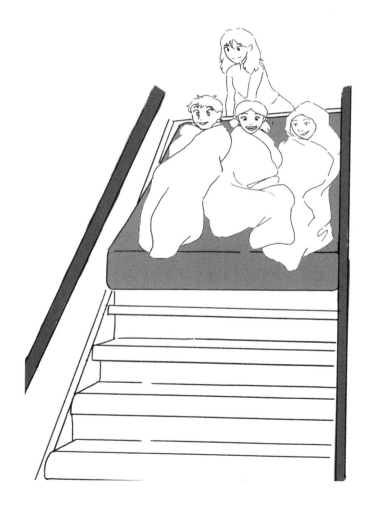

Lycra

I love Lycra so much my friends call me the "Lycra Princess." It's a crown I've been very proud to wear. I loved the idea of being a royal without as much responsibility as a queen. As I have aged and taken on more mentoring roles, I sometimes wonder if I need to upgrade my more mature position to the "Queen of Lycra." Because, like a queen, I have a sense of loyalty and duty to wrap the world in Lycra and help other therapists understand why it's so great.

I'm not at all bashful or apologetic about my love of Lycra. In consulting the Trauma Informed OT Facebook group, the response was an overwhelming "yes" when ask if a full section on Lycra would be helpful. So, here it is. I buy giant royal blue bolts in quantities of 100 meters from a wholesaler in California called Sportek. FM-65 Royal Blue is my favorite product and color. I use it for just about everything. For smaller amounts, I use The Stretch House in New York City. The important things to remember about buying Lycra is to ensure that it comes in four-way stretch. Many local sellers only have two-way stretch. When we view Lycra through the lens of neurology, the four-way stretch is necessary. Our sense of touch is incredibly specialized. There are individual neurons that will sense hot, cold, hair movement (like wind or quick movement), indentation for both sharp and dull objects, shearing forces, and more. When I think about sensory-related therapeutic input, three powerhouses are touch, proprioception, and vestibular input. Interoception is vital to "how we feel." But much of our interoceptive awareness is through the integration of our other senses, with these three still being powerhouses for how the brain interprets them. The brain calms with rhythm and repetition. Providing rhythmic taste, smell, and sight is a bit trickier. Of course, chewy foods are rhythmic, but that quality of "taste" is still registered through proprioception. While the brain is so complex and those networks overlap, I find the three powerhouses of proprioception, vestibular input, and touch are key to my therapeutic intervention. Lycra is my favorite modality because it targets each of them so beautifully, effortlessly, and relationally.

With a four-way stretch, the Lycra stimulates the stretch/sheer neuron receptors in our skin cells and provides awareness of how our body is moving. The firm and sturdy structure of the Sportex FM-65 provides stability for the joints that are involved in the contact with the fabric. Simply feeling Lycra as it is pulled around the body mimics our first relationally calm experience in the womb and stimulates our proprioceptive and tactile system in calm ways.

Typically, Lycra will also pull a person into a flexed movement pattern. As we look for therapeutic ways to move the body in our reflex integration activities, midline movement activities, and even vestibular movement activities, Lycra helps us facilitate these patterns. Sometimes, I want to give dual input to the brain by creating a little stress or risk while providing scaffolding for the client to gently expand their window of tolerance. When suspended, I can give the calming flexion and proprioceptive input along with rhythm while I stimulate the vestibular system through fast swinging. In this way, I have created a "just-right" challenge where I consider how the input is targeted towards the different neural receptors. I can challenge core muscles by suspending the Lycra and recreating the neurological feeling of when we were toddlers learning to walk. Supporting someone in a sheet of Lycra is an excellent way to respectfully and relevantly return to some of our earliest sensory inputs. One impactful therapy session I had was with an adoptive mom whose child struggled with caring touch. I invited Mom to sit in a bottom layer of Lycra and had her child sit in the layer above. We played a game of "guess my body part" through the Lycra. In the most beautiful interaction between the two of them, the child would snuggle up on top of the parent and offer safe touch to knees, elbows, shoulders, and eventually their nose and cheeks. As I watched this interaction, I was reminded of the joy I had when I carried my own children and lovingly caressed them through my belly.

While I don't practice any type of "re-birthing" scenario, I do see attachment benefits when a child pushes a ball through a long tube and greets the caregiver on the other end. A funny story about that activity is when I thought it would be fun to add big felt eyes to my tube of Lycra and pretend it was a snake. It was all fun and games until I had a child who thought of things in a very literal sense who became terrified that he was actually going to be eaten. Knowing your audience was the lesson I learned that day.

Some of the clients I work with don't feel seen or they feel overly exposed. For those who are older but feel unseen, I can place stickers in my Lycra layers and have them find them. We even play hide and seek within the layers ourselves. I make an intentional exclamation of "I see you!" when I find them. Just reflecting on these moments, I can feel the energy and therapeutic joy that is found in simply four layers of Lycra attached to stud boards in an old farmhouse living room.

For my clients who feel overly exposed, I've had great relational conversation success when I invite them to snuggle up with a weighted blanket or calming visual toy or scent and we just "hang out." Through the Lycra, I can still read their body language and see their outline. However, it is not face-to-face interaction, which can feel unsafe for so many of the clients I work with. I've had many parents leave a session like this completely shocked at how relationally verbal and connected their child (especially teens) can be with these sessions. Sometimes, "to get the ball rolling," I will invite them to toss a small ball back and forth and giggle a bit about how hard it is to hit an unseen target. When we blow bubbles, toss things together, or sip a similar beverage together, the words and emotions often bounce and spill out like the chosen therapeutic activity.

At $5/meter through the wholesalers, I can afford to gift large pieces of Lycra to my clients. For the majority of the people I work with who have experienced trauma or adversity, my presence, Lycra, a soft fuzzy bunny, bubbles, and a CapeAble weighted blanket are my go-to therapeutic tools. For anyone wanting more detailed visuals or video explanations, I have recorded an "All about Lycra" video on my podcast site, Martiot.podbean.com.

A colleague in Canada, Brendan McCann, OT, demonstrated a technique, similar to my Lycra nest swing mentioned above, that he calls a "teardrop swing," where he simply ties the corners into a point and suspends it with a carabiner from trees or other suspension supports.

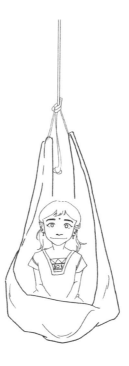

Another common Lycra creation that is available commercially is the body sock, or **silly sack**. If you have seen a decorative pillow cover with the hidden slit on the back side, that is similar in design to the ones I make. I use 1–3 meters of Lycra depending on the size of the child. I fold it lengthwise to form a long tube that is about three-quarters the height of the child. Since it will stretch, it does not need to be as tall as the child. I fold the tube so that the seam is in the middle as if looking at a hot dog bun. Next, I sew up the ends. To create a hole for the child to access the inside, I make a small cut that runs parallel to the end of the long seam on the opposite side. I used to leave an opening in that original long seam. However, I found that making a fresh cut on the opposite side rather than stopping and starting the seam means it is less likely to tear. When a child is seeking a lot of resistance in the silly sack, I add a metal ring to the top back of that long seam and attach a carabiner that I can then suspend while they run around the therapy space. To add the metal ring, I simply push some of the fabric through a single link of metal chain and then tie a knot, as if tying a balloon, on the side of the fabric that was pulled through.

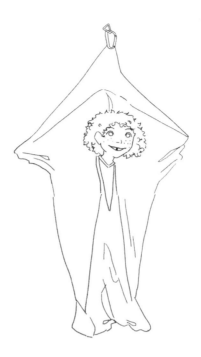

Once I discovered how to add the chain links to the Lycra in a secure fashion, it opened the possibility of my absolute favorite way to use Lycra, the **Lycra hammock cloud**. In my therapy space, this is my number-one tool. My clients *love* to be in my giant Lycra hammock cloud. I have several layers all connected to a single perimeter row of eye hooks screwed into the studs of three walls in my room. Since the remaining open side is fairly long, I have attached ropes that hang from eye hooks attached to the ceiling to provide more support along that side as well. Depending on the size and how many layers the client is suspended upon, the Lycra will suspend them at various heights. The more

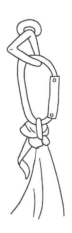

layers and lighter weight, the higher they will be towards the ceiling. For safety purposes, I use couch cushions, a foam mat, or a mattress at the entry point. Since gravity will pull the client towards the center of the material and studs are usually within a half-meter distance apart, I have never had a child fall out at a point near the wall. I do, however, still recommend close supervision. For many of my clients, this is a great proprioceptive and vestibular workout full of laughter and happy relational excitement. I have installed this system in every home I've lived in and it's a hit with my clients as well as neighborhood friends from birth to teenagers. Some caregivers enjoy it as well, especially since it promotes happy supported snuggles as their larger mass creates a soft dip in the gravitational pull that drives the child gleefully sliding towards them from the top edges.

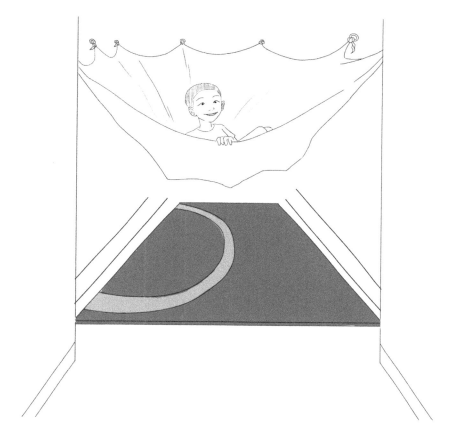

For a completely mobile and easy-to-use Lycra tool, a **1.5-meter piece** can be incredibly versatile. It can be held by two people to make a non-permanent Lycra hammock cloud. A knot could be tied on one corner and that could secure it in a door frame for one person to hold the other side, as if the person is in a stretchy boat.

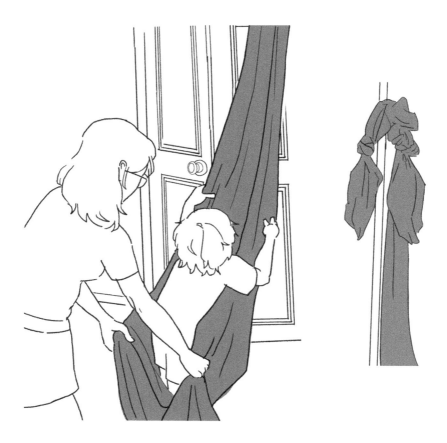

A wonderful activity to engage several people is to have one person pretend they are a tiny seed all balled up on the floor while several friends hold down the edges to cover them, supplying resistance to provide proprioception in a downward force. The person under the fabric then begins to push upwards as if they are a strong tree pushing branches through the "soil" towards the "sun." Sometimes I will press on the person and pretend to be the wind. I find this to be a gentle, respectful, and relevant way to begin to engage in safe touch activity for some of my most relationally tactile-adverse clients.

A **one-meter piece of Lycra** can even be used without any modification at all. I've had clients simply stretch it over their shoulders like a shawl or wrap it around themselves like a favorite blanket. I've added just one seam to form a loop of Lycra of various sizes to make stretch loop bands, tunnels, and compression tubes to slide over legs or the torso. In my therapeutic space, Lycra is one of my most powerful tools. It allows my clients to have independence over the amount of pressure they attain, and it is socially familiar and accessible.

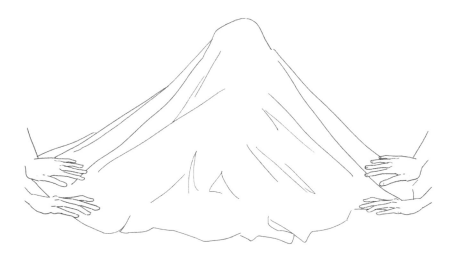

Bikes without pedals

Riding a bike is a complex activity. There are many steps and foundational skills involved. For some children, simply balancing requires an increased amount of practice. After seeing commercially available **balance bikes**, I wondered how to adapt a standard bike in an inexpensive way. I discovered removing the pedals is quite simple on most bikes. So now, rather than purchase them commercially, I find a bike with good tires at a secondhand store and simply remove the pedals to help the child gain practice scooting in a seated position while maintaining their balance as they glide down the sidewalk.

Yoga ball

A few years ago, I walked into a classroom and noticed a **store-bought exercise ball**. I asked the teacher why she didn't submit a request for purchase through the OT department that I could have bought her. She replied, "Well, I knew it would just get a pencil jabbed into it.

I figured it was cheaper to buy five of these than one of your expensive heavy-duty ones. Because there is nothing heavy-duty enough to prevent pencil jabs." I couldn't disagree. So I learned a valuable lesson from that teacher: I only buy "therapy balls" from discount stores. It really does ease the pocketbook pain when they don't last very long. Then, when they do pop, I cut the material into pieces and use it as a non-slip material, similar to the expensive commercial brand Dycem. I then use these pieces of deflated therapy ball to stabilize papers, line shelves, and create non-skid paths for sensory guidance.

Giant therapy balls are great for beginning a back-and-forth "serve and return" for children who find timing and ball-catching skills challenging. The bigger ball is easier to catch because the muscles can motor plan to connect with the large ball more easily. It also provides more proprioceptive feedback with its size and weight. Other uses include steam rolling it on top of the client, sitting for core strengthening, rhythmic bouncing, and an easy-target dodgeball session. Prone movement can even signal a reset to the vestibular system by rolling over the top while emphasizing the proprioceptive bump on the hands and feet.

Tactile spaces

When my clients have goals related to the tactile sense, I find that the more freedom and control I can give them, the more felt-safety they have. However, allowing someone who needs a lot of touch experience but does not have the awareness or integration to experience this tactile input in a controlled and tidy way can create chaos for even the most flexible therapist. While messes tend to not stress me, I know it can stress others. Plus, even I like messes that can be easily cleaned up. I'd rather spend an extra ten minutes setting the activity up for containment than spending an hour cleaning up when it gets widespread. My best example of failing at this concept was my seemingly brilliant and fun idea to pretend my own children and two of our neighbor friends were ninja board breakers. We had recently installed a bathroom vanity and there were various thickness sheets of Styrofoam that were used for packaging of the large cabinets. I would hold the pieces up and they would kick and arm-chop them with confidence and delight. About five minutes in, I realized things were getting a little messier than I had originally envisioned. Not wanting to ruin the momentum of the fun, I decided I would invest the time after the completion and simply let the children continue to have their fun. Well, 45 minutes later, my children were making snow angels and tossing the tiny little beads up in the air as if it was snowing in our dining room. It seemed the entire room had transformed into a white snow globe. I was clearly in over my capacity to clean this up efficiently, especially as the static electricity began taking effect and the foam beads began crawling up the walls and into the shutters.

In a moment of "this was a *much* better idea in my head," I decided my only option to rein this mess in was a leaf blower. In my head, I thought the force of the air would be enough to blow the tiny bits into a manageable pile. Once that idea came to life outside of my head, I realized it was doing the opposite and blowing things higher up the walls and more finely dispersed. At this point, the children were squealing with more delight than I have ever heard prior or since. I went down the arousal continuum myself into complete dissociation and simply handed the electric leaf blower to the five-year-old. I can't even really say "the rest is history" because I'm *still* finding tiny Styrofoam beads *everywhere*. I even moved houses. Yet I still find them in a pair of shoes, the back of a photo, inside a box of crayons, even in the small grooves on the back of LEGO® bricks. It is to date my most epic tactile sensory fail. So I've learned to be better about containing those messes. I'll share a few of my favorite mess containers here.

Sewn sweatshirt

When I taught my class "OT and PT on a Shoestring Budget," I would ask therapists for their tried-and-true tips. A lot of their brilliant suggestions were about how to transport equipment or keep things more neat and tidy than my previously mentioned styrofoam chaos party. One of the therapists taught me this great flexible and mobile way to carry around her rice, bean, or corn sensory bins without them spilling in her trunk or having them thrown across the room by eager tactile explorers.

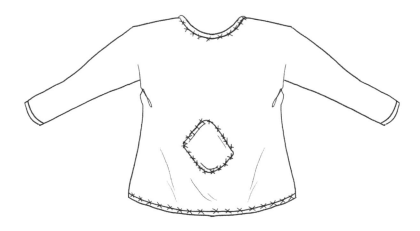

The first step is to sew the collar and the waist of a sweatshirt shut. If you don't sew, I've had success closing them with fabric glue and even a stapler when I worked in schools. Once those openings are closed, the cuffs of the sleeves are the only openings. Next, put the rice, beans, corn, or any dry tactile material inside the belly of the shirt, using the sleeves as the entry. Sometimes I will hide other things inside the material to work on stereognosis (the ability to identify a three-dimensional object by touch without using your sense of sight). I've had a therapist tell me that she cut a hole in the belly and glued in a piece of flexible vinyl so that there was a "window" to see the contents inside. Finally, when the child puts their hands in through the sleeves, the sleeves create a tight tube that prevents them from quickly removing too much material and throwing it around. They can feel the contents inside of the shirt container while keeping it very contained in a flexible material that molds to their lap if needed. Sometimes the commonly used plastic storage bins can be accidentally dumped over since they are rigid. When the child is finished with the activity in the sweatshirt, the arms can be tied together like the first knot of shoe tying. This prevents any of the material from flowing out during transportation. Once I learned of this homemade hack, I never used a "sensory bin" for dry stimuli again. If this seems too complicated, I recently heard of putting a Quaker oatmeal container inside the foot part of a long sock. This provides a stiff container area for the sensory material while the sock acts similar to the sleeve, limiting the amount of material available for tossing around the room or rubbing into the carpet.

Camping tent

When I want the child to have a fuller-body tactile experience such as the ball pit or larger containers of corn, I place a child-sized plastic pool or other bin that would fit their body inside a camping tent. When I zip up the door, the child is free to toss the contents around and fully experience the sensations while keeping the material contained within the walls of the tent. Most tents have screens that can be used to keep a watchful eye on the child while also facilitating relational connection as the child is inside and the caregiver might be outside.

Fitted sheets

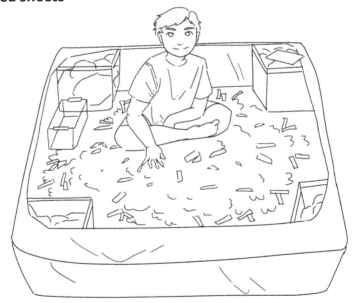

My son is an avid LEGO builder. If you've collected more than a few sets, you may understand the idea that the best creations come from the ability to spread the pieces out on the floor and sit among them. In an effort to contain the sprawl of foot-pain-inducing lost pieces, we discovered a creative strategy. We place the bins that hold the LEGO pieces in the four corners of a fitted bed sheet. Then, we dump the individual pieces onto the sheet. With the correct-sized bins, it creates a nest the size of a mattress for my son to sit inside with walls to minimize the sprawl. For the clients with less propensity to propel pieces, this is an excellent and inexpensive way to be submerged in a dry texture that assists with ease of clean-up upon completion.

Cotton balls with scents

I often use scented items to explore what helps my clients feel safe and comfortable or energized and activated. I have a variety of lotions, soaps, foods, and candles that I use regularly. For some clients, I need to make the scent more accessible without being long-lasting. Lotions and soaps can sometimes continue to stimulate due to their liquid nature and being absorbed into skin and clothing. To solve this issue, a therapist in one of my courses recommended putting the scent into a cotton ball. The cotton ball then absorbs the moisture to keep it more contained. She then further suggested that the cotton ball be placed in a container that could be squeezed to release air. An example would be a condiment bottle or a squirt bottle. When the olfactory stimulus is desired, the therapist simply squeezes the bottle and then scent travels out attached to the air molecules. But it is short-lasting and leaves no lingering residue once the stimulation is ceased.

Baoding balls

I like the soft, melodic sound of baoding relaxation balls. I often pick them up in Chinatown when I visit New York. They are great for in-hand manipulation exercises, rolling around the palm, and rhythmic auditory and visual stimulation. I love all the different patterns, designs, and colors, and how they are often packaged in a fancy silk box. While I need to be mindful of them being thrown since they are metal, most of my clients are happy to hold them in their hands. They have an inherent calming rhythm and can be shaken a little harder to match a slightly more activated system. Egg shakers are another nice auditory option for shaking sounds. I love the variety of Easter eggs available in the spring. When I see unique colors or characters like bunnies, baseballs, dinosaurs, etc., I try to buy a few. This way, I have a variety of choices that help my clients' interests be represented. Once they choose their eggs, they can next choose what to fill them with. Rice, beans, sand, flour, jingle bells, and pebbles all make very distinct sounds in a taped-up plastic egg.

Electric toothbrushes

Vibration is a type of touch sensation that is interpreted by unique neurons that differ from those that detect pain, itch, and light touch. Because of the way vibration is interpreted, it can be a way to desensitize the body and increase the sense of safety. Weary parents have long used the trick of a buggy or car ride to soothe a crying infant. Vibrating pillows and handheld therapeutic massage tools have become increasingly common as people seek ways to relieve stress. A commercially available product called a Z-Vibe is used by many therapists to provide vibratory input to the mouth. I find them to be very effective clinically. But they can be cost-prohibitive for some families that I work with. So I substitute them with electric toothbrushes. Not all electric toothbrushes vibrate at the same frequency. Different clients also prefer different frequencies of stimulation. Because of this, I buy a few to have on hand in my therapy supplies so that people can try them before they buy them. Most of my clients prefer the Spinbrush or Oral B brands of electric toothbrushes. I use these as a pre-feeding stimulation before introducing new or complex textured foods. I also use them to simply hold in the hands or on the feet before therapeutic tactile activities for my clients who tend to be more sensitive in those areas. I've even had success putting one under a pillow for a more diffuse stimulation.

Stacking cups

When my children were young, I discovered a multitude of uses for stacking cups. Because of this, I keep a stack of small plastic cups readily available in my therapy space and use them often. I can sort things into them or pour things out of them. They are great for wrist rotation and dexterity as you stack them upside down or drinking rim side up. My clients make large stacking cup towers and squeal with delights as they run the swing into them, watching the stacked cups crash to the ground. This activity is illustrated on the cover of this book. We use them as obstacle course markers and targets to reach for when crossing midline on a bolster swing. If they are different colors, they become easy sortable objects or items to be picked up in a sequence as we work on increasing the ability to follow multiple-step requests. Sometimes, we even use them to hydrate by filling them with water to drink.

Vegetable brushes

When I think of tactile stimulation, I do believe that surgical scrub brushes provide a lot of great therapeutic benefits. While looking online to buy them in bulk one day, I found a similar product in really fun colors marketed as vegetable brushes. I bought a few to test out and discovered they are incredibly similar. The added benefit of the colors is the interest and increased motivation for some of my younger clients to engage in the repetitive skin-deep pressure stimulation that I recommend with the brushes. I also like that I can have different colors to offer choices, because something as simple as providing a choice is a hallmark of trauma-responsive care. Color also makes me happy, and I feel like it makes others happy too.

Sensitive-skin shaving cream

Vegetable brushes, feathers, various cloth textures, and the soft fur of our farm animals are some of my favorite dry-texture therapeutic activities. For a more intense wet experience, I use sensitive-skin Gillette shaving cream. I like this brand and type because it has less odor than others I have tried. For clients who have both smell and tactile aversions, sometimes the cheaper and stronger-scented products are simply too much stimulation for them to process. I use the shaving cream in a progressive exposure sequence depending on where I assess the child will have the just-right challenge. I want them to be mildly uncomfortable and moving towards the alert column of the arousal continuum without pushing them into alarm. For some clients, this means beginning with the shaving cream in a closed Ziplock bag. To bring interest, I add a drop of color (powdered paint, liquid paint, or food coloring). I allow the child to become accustomed to the activity within the bounds of non-direct-touch safety. Maybe towards the end, I will increase the risk by cutting a small snip off the corner of the bag to make it a piping activity. They can interact with the texture without actually touching it. Some days, this is where we stop. Some days, this is where we start and then they are invited, but never forced, to put one finger in. Then maybe I hide something of interest that they must transfer from a bucket of shaving cream to a bucket of water that will wash off the soapy texture quickly to provide for that very small dose of perceived discomfort. An effective strategy I have instilled in my practice is to provide a "safety rag." This is a hand towel that is wet on one end and dry on the other. Any time a client gets past their comfort zone with the shaving cream, they can immediately be brought back to their safety by cleaning off the tactile input quickly. This has been highly effective with even my most tactile-hesitant clients.

If my client is wanting to feel the entire can of shaving cream in one sitting, I provide structure and non-judgmental boundaries for that experience. I ask that parents send the child in swim clothes, and we use large containers. Since I have access to a bathroom, we often use the tub. Children's inflatable swim pools and, for smaller children, even large storage containers outside work well. If the therapy space is not conducive to this, I encourage the parents to allow the child an entire can at home. Since shaving cream is soap, this can be a fun bathtime replacement on occasion. I find when children pursue this much stimulation, it helps to allow them to fully immerse themselves and have extra time to explore and experiment. What happens when we add different textures like sticky syrup to the soap? Do you like mixing colors? Do you delight in me getting a bit on my own body and we share giggles and quick eye gazes as I make silly noises and faces to show how I feel about the texture? Can we talk about how it feels on my skin as compared to theirs? How can we use this over-the-top experience to connect relationally?

CapeAble weighted products

I met the founder and inventor of the CapeAble weighted blankets, Marna Pacheco, at a conference. Before meeting Marna, I made my own weighted products. I would buy stuffed animals and replace the cotton stuffing with plastic beads from the craft stores. I would use those same little plastic beads and attempt to make my own weighted blankets and lap pads. If you have ever made your own weighted products, you are likely aware of how difficult it is to sew those channels without breaking your needles or making your lines look like the waves of a rainy day at the beach. Straight, evenly distributed channels are not easy, especially when you don't want the beads inside to move around a lot. Marna makes this seem easy. She has invented a special machine that takes care of all of that and combines it with beautiful and feel-great fabrics. I love that the beads in her blankets don't slide around. She has done great research on how the skin receptors being hit by a constant and conformed contact makes sure that the neurons can sense them evenly for better integration on the somatosensory cortex level. Simply put, even though this is a chapter on how to make your own equipment, I don't make my own weighted blankets. Because Marna has perfected the therapeutic weighted blanket for me, I recommend them any chance I get (www.capeable.com).

Auditory equipment

I do use professional auditory programs and specific interventions in my own therapy space. But I also add other creative ways to stimulate the sense of sound. I love to experiment with food storage containers, pots and pans, and even items in the recycling container bins. I find many of my clients have difficulty with pressure modulation and I've had several expensive drum mallets break. I find wooden spoons to be very sturdy and easily replaced. I also love the creative flexibility we can have when we discuss and become curious about how different textures and materials feel and sound when activated in a drum-like manner.

My iPhone is my most used auditory tool. I have downloaded files of therapeutic music, the EASe Listening Therapy app from Audioforge, where I can customize modifications, and Spotify playlists of low-tempo and fast-tempo music. As I get to know my clients and their preferences, I can even customize a few songs into a playlist specifically with them. I find the simple curiosity of "What kind of music do you like?" or "What is your favorite song?" can be a great way to build rapport with my clients. I often see delight when they walk in the room and I pull up a playlist of songs we chose together during their last session as they self-regulated on one of my swings. To hear "your song" as you enter a space can be a powerful way to feel "seen" and "heard."

Visual equipment
Pool lights/orbs
I enjoy looking at pictures of sensory spaces full of string lights. However, I need to be mindful and aware of my clients using strings as a self-harm weapon. Yet I love when I can turn off the lights and my clients snuggle up in the Lycra hammock with a focused light object. I found little light-up floating pool orbs at a market store one time and they are perfect. They can be sanitized because they are waterproof, and they usually have a pleasing texture. During seasonal holidays, I try to keep an eye out for little battery-operated items that change color. I use them often as night lights. When they slowly change color, they make great visual focus "fidgets."

Finger lights
Finger lights are an inexpensive and fun way to work on eye–hand coordination, fine motor skills, eye tracking, attention, and motor planning. I like the little colored lights that can be found in the party favor aisle where a little rubber band secures a tiny colored light to each finger. I find that these lights can be used on the hand or even hidden around the therapy space for an interesting "hide and seek" in the dark. As I learned about the neuroanatomy of the sense of vision, I saw that the eyes are anatomically structured to be on a higher threat response in the dark. Some of my clients tend to be in this high threat response habitually. So when I meet them in that moment and engage them in a fun, connected, playful, rewarding game, I can begin to build new neural connections that help decrease that threat

response default. I can use playful colorful lights to pair that threat sensation with relational connection and my protection.

Colored plastic films

I use flashlights and other battery-operated lights to influence the sensory environment. In addition to brightness, color can be fun and enlightening when exploring how various sensations influence how a person is feeling. Gift wrap, report covers, and other thin plastics can provide inexpensive ways to change the color of lights. Some clinics even purchase ready-made colored covers for overhead lights. One of the organizations I consulted with used covers that looked like a beautiful blue sky and big puffy white clouds as part of their TBRI sensory-mindful redecoration.

Small resin farm animals

When I taught at the Florida Elks group last year, we were each asked to show and tell our favorite therapy tool. One of the therapists mentioned "small resin animals miniatures" from Amazon. I, of course, was curious about these since I work in a farm environment. I ordered them for $13 and have been incredibly pleased at the diversity these have provided. We sort them, match them, and hide them. They do well in the putty as well as hidden under small drinking cups. We can create stories about them and talk about the sounds and smells the animals they represent make. We can create families with them and talk about how families often look different from each other. We can pretend they have personalities. Sometimes, I simply hand a handful of them to my client and ask, "What shall we do with these?" So often, I learn something about my client from playing with these animals that they would likely not feel safe to talk about in regard to their own feelings. But they will talk about it from the animal's perspective, which is often very similar to their own. This can open pivotal doors to their guarded thoughts.

Chart stickers

As a school therapist, I spent a lot of time thinking about how to improve spacing when working with handwriting. I found the little stickers for behavior charts were the perfect size. They were also cheap and easily transported—two important things to consider. While I purchased them for handwriting spacing, I quickly found that they were useful for so many other things. They provided a good target for visual scanning, foot placement, and cueing to go to the next paragraph when reading. Most kids love them. In my therapy space at the farm, I stick them in the layers of my Lycra hammock cloud to be climbed through and located by eager clients. I place them on my face to encourage eye contact. I understand how trauma can make eye contact uncomfortable for many of my clients, so even looking in the direction of my face can be relational progress for them. In the TBRI training, one of the activities we teach to promote compassion and empathy is the Band-Aid game. The premise is that we share our hurts and put Band-Aids on each other. It's a beautiful way to connect with one another and I've seen great progress. This is one reason I have a fun collection of Band-Aids in my own space to share with my clients. When a client is not ready for the full Band-Aid analogy, we can start with tiny chart stickers to simply bring visual awareness to various body parts in fun, engaging, and non-threatening ways. For any interaction involving sticking something to a client, I encourage them to have full autonomy and consent for that touch activity.

Balloons

Balloons are other essentials for my therapy bag. For a client who needs more time to motor plan, a balloon is a lightweight choice that moves through the air more slowly than most playground balls. It also hurts less when it bumps into someone, whether intentional or not. Robyn Gobbel talks a lot about "serve and return" with the pattern of connection and attachment. Literally serving and returning a balloon can be great practice for taking turns in conversations and other relational moments. When a client is proficient with the balloon toss and the therapist wants to increase the challenge a bit, two of my favorite strategies are marbles inside or tape on the outside. Even one marble will shift the center of gravity in the balloon and create a less predictable wobble as it is tossed back and forth. This small amount of unpredictability can help create resilience when done in a playful manner. When tape is placed on one side, the balloon will default to falling towards that extra weighted side. This can add an element of predictable balloon course change challenge.

Tape

Tape is another common item that I like to have on hand. I use it to hold things together, label things, and create visual borders. I've made obstacle courses and "tightropes" on the floor. We can use it to measure how far someone jumps or indicate a boundary that the client can perceive as a "safe zone." I've even had success with a few of my teens who pick at their skin. Some mention that the sensation of pulling the tape off their arms, legs, and hands can be satisfying and decrease the amount of injurious picking.

Taste activities

Jelly Belly beans

While I try to be mindful of nutrition, I also want to have fun with my clients. After all, I only have two rules in my therapy space: "Have fun" and "Stop." Every child who enters my room is greeted with a level of enthusiasm I perceive will be tolerated by assessing their body language. One of the very first things I tell them is these two rules. I assure them I want us both to have a great time. Then I let them know that we can both use a safety word, "Stop." I will only use it if I perceive them to be in harm's way. They are allowed to use it for any activity I request of them that they don't want to do. It's a way to give them perceived control right from the get-go. I do mention that just because we stop in that moment, it doesn't mean we won't "go" another time. But when we do, I will be sure they feel secure, safe, and successful. Trauma informed means making accommodations for felt-safety. Part of "have fun" is tiny jelly beans. I like to have a constant supply of both regular gustatorily pleasing and predictable types as well as the gross-tasting BeanBoozled game variety. For many of my clients with food goals, I find these little beans to be a minimal sugar investment with a large potential reward of trying different tastes. I allow them the control of spitting out the flavors they don't like. I try to mix in known and preferred tastes. Jelly Belly beans are such a delightful way to incorporate slight dysregulation within a fun context of connection and relationship. Food can be so connecting and evoke feelings of vulnerability. For some of my clients, this is their first experience of being able to share their adversity. A simple "Ew! This was so gross! Here—try it!" is a very natural communication rhythm. When they invite me into this dysregulation, it is a powerful way for me to convey to them "I see you. I'm with you. I will do hard things *with* you." As much as I'm against filling kids with sugar, I'm pretty open to Jelly Belly games.

Frozen Tootsie Rolls

Another sweet treat I allow in my therapy space is frozen chewy candy (I use Tootsie Rolls) and frozen liquorice sticks. Both are highly motivating for most kids, and freezing them really changes the texture and oral motor skill required to consume them. For kids who don't eat meat, I can be curious about whether they reject chewy proteins because they get muscle fatigue in their mouth. Most children eagerly accept frozen candy. When they reject it after it doesn't break apart easily, that is data for me to wonder if their jaws are easily fatigued.

Other therapeutic activities

Daily activities and routines

The best way to make new habits and neural connections is through small exposures or experiences over time. Dr. Perry refers to this pattern as "dosing" (Perry & Winfrey, 2021, p. 111; Perry, 2021). Since the relaxed or alert but not fearful brain tends to "check in and check out" multiple times a minute, rehabilitation works with that pattern. We practice a little bit throughout the day for a better outcome than a solid hour once a week. Because of this, I try whenever possible to incorporate new therapeutic moments during daily activities and routines. Cracking 15 eggs to make a giant scramble is helpful in a treatment session. But cracking two eggs each morning and allowing that learning to integrate over a week is even more powerful. Giving a child choices throughout the day is more effective than me bombarding them with decisions in the hour that I have them. We need time for subconscious integration.

We also need time for repairs. No one can be perfect all the time.

Even the best parenting strategies are bound to fail from time to time. It is the ability to apologize and figure out a way forward that builds a truly strong foundation. With this in mind, I try to help caregivers set up their homes for sensory-rich exploration and opportunity for many small therapeutic sensations. When possible, I add components of relationship and connection to the moments. For example, when you make a special recipe, call the person that passed it down to you or share the emotional connection to it while you make it.

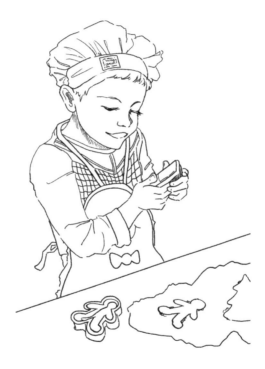

Use familiar items like couch pillows to make forts and encourage something new, such as reading a new story or playing a new game. This pairs the newness of the story or game with being surrounded by familiar items. Pitch a camping tent in the living room. Sometimes people who have experienced adversity have difficulty feeling safe when there is too much novelty. Camping in a familiar home may feel safer than hours away in a completely different sensory environment. With people who crave control and familiarity, I try to tether a piece of past perceived safety to new therapeutic experiences. I try to build off skills they feel confident in as I grow them into new accomplishments. I use their daily patterns and familiar activities to form the foundation while I "dose" them with my therapeutic suggestions.

Nature

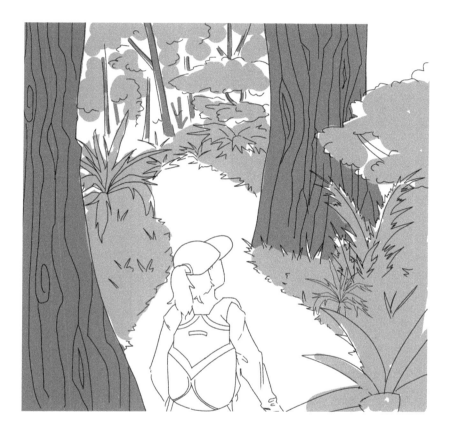

All living things do better with sunshine and water. My own children often had their bathtime before dinner, around that 4pm hour of too tired to be cheerful but too early to eat supper and go to bed. Countless studies point to nature and green spaces being good for our bodies and souls. Working on a farm, it's easy for me to incorporate nature in my sessions. But I don't always utilize the full farm space. Sometimes I bring a single potted plant inside or ask the client to do an outdoor scavenger hunt and bring me things that feel good to them or that they simply want to share with me. I encourage caregivers to take little day trips to parks and other nature areas close to their homes. I encourage them to find grass, take off their shoes, and simply sit still in the green space. I encourage the caregiver to view outdoors much like we approached the shaving cream—with curiosity and sequential exposure. How does it feel to sit in a sunbeam by the window at different times of the day? Are there any places nearby where there is movement of water? What noises do you hear outside? What do we think about those noises? Can we make a trip to the grocery store a sensory experience? Can we explore a farmers' market? How can I work within my client's financial budget, community, and location resources to encourage them to get outside? This is such an important part of my treatment plan.

Simple Sparrow Sequential Relational Path

In 2018, a friend named Trudy approached me about making a path for a children's home in Colombia. She wanted something similar to videos found on the internet by searching for sensory paths, but with more intention and neurological and trauma awareness. So many of the paths Trudy was seeing available commercially seemed so haphazard with their colors and movements. Having a child jump and spin at the end and then asking them to sit still or have a conversation goes against the current science of how movement influences our neurology and arousal state. Thus, the Simple Sparrow Sequential Relational Path was developed. Trudy brought understanding of the relational and cultural aspects, Jamie Tanner created the beautiful artwork, and I thought through the sensory and neurologically stimulating elements. Our path is unique because it guides the participants through sequential exercises and movements designed to influence neural networks while also creating an attachment and relationally rich experience.

The path has two mirrored paths so that the participants are doing the same types of movements in synchrony. One side is intentionally less active for participants who may not want to be as quick or intense with their movement. But they are still mirrored. For example, while one participant is jumping and spinning from each portion of the honeycomb, the other is slowly rotating and stepping through the sunflowers. This portion of the path is rich with jagged, sharp lines and bright activating colors in yellows and oranges to match a higher energy level of a client while the therapist or caregiver begins to co-regulate with them through their mirror neurons and matched rhythmic repetitive movements. This portion of the path is the activation of the brainstem and diencephalon. Past the activations portion is a "midline vine" which invites the participants to cross their feet past their midline in a cross-weaving pattern as the movements engage both sides of the brain by crossing the midline and landing with a proprioceptive step. The colors are neutral and nature colors of greens and browns. This portion of the path is the activation of the midbrain and limbic structures. The last portion of the path is the frog poses and logs. The frog poses continue to encourage movement patterns that engage the limbic structures and facilitate more proprioceptive input as the participants bend forward and press into the ground with the illustrated movement suggestions. The blues and greens and smooth visual lines begin to calm the nervous system. All the while on the path, participants are connecting, relating, and mirroring one another. The final stage of the brown logs invites the participants to engage in a frontal-cortex-stimulating activity of conversation. The questions are intended to invite connection and relationship. While the path is available for purchase on the Simple Sparrow farm website (www. simplesparrow.farm), it is my hope that this section helps give a better understanding of intentionality when creating a sensory space. A sample of the Simple Sparrow path can be seen on the cover of this book. For a deeper explanation of how various sensory inputs affects our arousal and activation, please see my first book, *The Connected Therapist: Relating Through the Senses*.

Therapeutic use of self

The therapist's or caregiver's body movements, co-regulation, tone of voice, acceptance, and other ways we bring our full being to the treatment space are therapeutic use of self. Simply providing a safe, inclusive, welcoming environment is therapy. I once worked with a teen who experienced severe childhood trauma. Their caregiver had tried many well-intended counselors who invited them to talk, but that led to further dissociation and shutdown for the teen. Our first session, we simply made waffles from a mix. I began with empowerment and meeting physical needs. The focus was on food infused with community. While the teen was engaged and experiencing safety without pressure, I was able to notice body language, multi-step processing (or lack thereof), eye contact, how many times they "checked out" or dissociated, and even oral motor and table skills. When we first built a foundation of safety, we were able to simply sit on a swing and blow bubbles for Daisy dog.

Now we had moved into the rhythmic back and forth of communication and relationship. As this became comfortable, I asked if I could sit close enough to the swing that they would occasionally bump into me, making safe/deep-touch physical contact with my body. This playful physical contact then led me to a path of being able to talk about how my body responds to sensation so that we could explore how their body responded to various sensations. From there, we were able to identify sensory-based experiences that the caregiver could use to help them self-regulate when things at home became overwhelming for them. But in the beginning, it was less about the activity and more about simply using my body to help them tolerate another human and trust that I would not harm them.

While we cooked, I made sure to not block them in. I used rhythm in my voice and was curious and playful with my tone. Did they respond better to a higher pitch that matched their delayed developmental age? Or did I need to bring it down a bit to be a deeper resonation because of auditory preference? Could they tolerate bumping into my arm if I reached past them to get them tools for cooking? I considered all these things and was then better able to adjust the way the caregiver and I interacted with them. I used my own body language, movements, even my appearance to guide them to a felt-safety. I pulled back hair so they could easily scan my face for non-verbal intent, wore soft clothing without a lot of visually distracting patterns, and was conscious about my own hygiene to prevent sensitivity to body odor.

While I used insurance codes for therapeutic activity based on the cooking activity, the actual change during those first two sessions was more influenced by how I brought myself to that session. I hope to encourage anyone reading this book to know that *you* truly are the most effective "therapy." I hope this book has inspired you to bring yourself to the session with new practical suggestions filled with compassion, optimism, and excitement. I hope this book inspires you to simply be present in the moment, patiently waiting for connection, and full of adoration for any human in your presence. As many OTs like to say, "If it works, it's treatment; if not, it's assessment!" Remember too that those little changes, like simply giving someone more time, compassion, and the benefit of the doubt can make big differences. I also lean heavily into a principle of hope. I believe there is always hope.

References

Anda, R. F., Felitti, V. J., Bremner, J. D., Walker, J. D., *et al*. (2006). The enduring effects of abuse and related adverse experiences in childhood: A con-
vergence of evidence from neurobiology and epidemiology. *European
Archives of Psychiatry and Clinical Neuroscience, 256,* 174–186.

Barrett, L. F. (2017). *How Emotions are Made: The Secret Life of the Brain.* New
York, NY: Houghton Mifflin Harcourt.

Daishonin, N. (n.d.). *The Writings of Nichiren Daishonin.* Volume II. www.
nichirenlibrary.org/en/wnd-2/Content/372

Douglas, A. C., M.S. (2021). Meeting Children Where They Are: The Neurosequential Model of Therapeutics. NCFA (National Council for Adoption).
https://adoptioncouncil.org/publications/meeting-children-where-they-
are-the-neurosequential-model-of-therapeutics

Felitti, V. J., Anda, R. F., Nordenberg, D., Williamson, D. F. *et al*. (1998). Relationship of childhood abuse and household dysfunction to many of the
leading causes of death in adults: The Adverse Childhoood Experiences
(ACE) Study. *American Journal of Preventive Medicine 14,* 4, 245–258.

Garner, S., & Perry, B. D. (2023). *Translating the Six R's for the Educational*
Setting. Revised and updated from *A '6Rs" Translation Template for* Educators, 2020). NMN Press, Houston.

Gobbel, R. (n.d.). Being With. https://robyngobbel.com/beingwith

Gobbel, R. (2021). Ep. 27: Marti Smith on becoming a connected therapist.
The Baffling Behavior Show [Parenting after Trauma]. https://podcasts.
apple.com/us/podcast/parenting-after-trauma-with-robyn-gobbel/
id1543535062?i=1000517935398

Gobbel, R. (2023). *Raising Kids with Big, Baffling Behaviors: Brain-Body-Sensory
Strategies That Really Work.* London: Jessica Kingsley Publishers.

Gray, C. (2000). *The New Social Stories Book.* Arlington, TX: Future Horizon.

Greene, R. W. (2021). *The Explosive Child [Sixth Edition]: A New Approach for
Understanding and Parenting Easily Frustrated, Chronically Inflexible Children.* New York, NY: HarperCollins Publishers.

Mateos, P. & Rodríguez, A. (2021, September 20). The Hebb Synapse before Hebb: Theories of synaptic function in learning and memory before Hebb (1949), with a discussion of the long-lost synaptic theory of William McDougall. *Frontiers in Behavioral Neuroscience*. www.frontiersin.org/articles/10.3389/fnbeh.2021.732195/full.

Perry, B. D. (n.d.). The Neurosequential Network. NMT™. www.neurosequential.com/nmt.

Perry, B. D. (2001). *The Neurodevelopmental Impact of Violence in Childhood*. In D. Schetky & E. P. Benedek (Eds) *Textbook of Child and Adolescent Forensic Psychiatry*. (pp. 221–238). Washington, D.C: American Psychiatric Press.

Perry, B. D. (2006). *Applying Principles of Neurodevelopment to Clinical Work with Maltreated and Traumatized Children: The Neurosequential Model of Therapeutics*. In N. B. Webb (Ed) *Working with Traumatized Youth in Child Welfare*. (Chapter 3). New York, NY: The Guilford Press.

Perry, B. D. (2009). Examining Child Maltreatment Through a Neurodevelopmental Lens: Clinical Applications of the Neurosequential Model of Therapeutics. *Journal of Loss and Trauma*, 14, 4, 240–255.

Perry, B.D. (2013). *The Neurosequential Model of Therapeutic in Young Children*. In K. Brandt, B.D. Perry, S. Seligman, & E. Tronick (Eds) *Infant and Early Childhood Mental Health*. (pp. 21–47). New York, NY: American Psychiatric Press.

Perry, B. D. (2020). *The Neurosequential Model: a developmentally sensitive, neuroscience-informed approach to clinical problem solving*. In J. Mitchell, J. Tucci, & E. Tronick (Eds) *The Handbook of Therapeutic Child Care for Children*. (pp. 137 - 155) London: Jessica Kingsley Publishers.

Perry, B. D. (2021, June). *Keynote Presentation* [Lecture]. Rising Tide Conference, Danville, IL.

Perry, B. D. & Hambrick E. P. (2008). The Neurosequential Model of Therapeutics. *Reclaiming Children and Youth*, 17, 3, 38–43.

Perry, B. D., Pollard, R. A., Blakley, T. L., Baker, W. L., & Vigilante, D. (1995). Childhood Trauma, the Neurobiology of Adaptation and "Use-dependent" Development of the Brain: How "States" Become "Traits". *Infant Mental Health Journal*, 16, 4.

Perry, B. D. & Szalavitz, M. (2017). *The Boy Who was Raised as a Dog* [*Third Edition*]. New York, NY: Basic Books.

Perry, B. D., & Winfrey, O. (2021). *What Happened to You? Conversations on Trauma, Resilience, and Healing*. New York, NY: Flatiron Books.

Porges, S. W. (2011). *The Polyvagal Theory: Neurophysiological Foundations of Emotions, Attachment Communication, Self-Regulation*. New York, NY: W.W. Norton.

Porges, S. W. (2017). *The Pocket Guide to the Polyvagal Theory: The Transformative Power of Feeling Safe*. New York, NY W.W. Norton.

Purvis, K. B., Cross, D. R., & Sunshine, W. L. (2007). *The Connected Child: Bring Hope and Healing to Your Adoptive Family*. New York, NY: McGraw-Hill Education.

Smith, M. (2021). *The Connected Therapist: Relating Through the Senses* (J. Tanner, Illus.). Austin, TX: Marti Smith Seminars.

Smith, M., & Smith, R. (n.d.). *Kalmar App*. htttp://kalmar.creativetherapies. com

Stackhouse, T. (2022). [Personal interview by the author].

Stackhouse, T., MacInnes, S., & Maunder, M. (n.d.). SpIRiTed Conversations. https://www.spiritedconversationspodcast.com

TCU. (n.d.). *Karyn Purvis Institute of Child Development* [YouTube Channel]. YouTube. Accessed 19 Oct 2023 from https://www.youtube.com/@karynpurvisinstituteofchil8864/videos

Van der Kolk, B. (2014). *The Body Keeps the Score: Brain, Mind, and Body in the Healing of Trauma*. New York, NY: Penguin.

Weber, J. D., Whiting, D., Erickson, C., & Stackhouse, T. (2023). *Mindfulness and Me—Webinar Replay, with Tracy Murnan Stackhouse* [Webinar]. The National Fragile X Foundation.

Index

"A" functions 32
activity analysis 13–17, 29
Alliance of Trauma Responsive OT
    Practitioners (A-TROT) 156
amygdala 105
assessments
    foundational questions 147–9
    initial interactions 149–52
    matching expectations 152–6
auditory equipment 188–9
autoimmune issues 52–4

balance bikes 179
balloons 191–2
baoding relaxation balls 184–5
Barrett, Lisa Feldman 24
"Being With" presence 15
Body Keeps the Score, The (van
    der Kolk) 53, 120
Born for Love (Perry) 11
Boy Who Was Raised as a
    Dog, The (Perry) 11
brain regions
    and activity analysis 29
    air traffic control analogy
        for 24–8, 29–30
    developmental sequences in 30
    rehabilitation of 27–8
    and resilience 28–8
    spider's web metaphor for 30
brainstem
    air traffic control analogy for 31–2
    autoimmune issues 52–4

breathing 47–50
    difficulties with food 35–42
    muscular eye movements 54–7
    functions of 31–5
    heart rate normalization 43–5
    temperature regulation 45–7
    weight and nutrition 50–2
breathing 47–50
Brown, Brené 78

camping tent 183
CapeAble weighted products 188
caregivers
    and co-regulation 9–10
    and treatment planning 163–5
cerebellum
    engagement 71–9
    fine motor skills 68–71
    functions of 58–9
    gross motor skills 62–8
    sensory integrative processing
        79–103
    sleep 59–62
chart stickers 190–1
co-regulation
    and caregivers 9–10
    and state-dependent functioning 20
colored plastic film 190
communication (verbal and
    non-verbal) 128–31
Connected Therapist, The:
    Relating Through the Senses
    (Smith) 82–3, 130

cortex
  communication (verbal and
    non-verbal) 128–31
  functions of 127–8
  sense of time 131–3
  waiting ability 131–3
Cross, D. R. 9

daily activities and routines 193–5
Daishonin, Nichiren 10
delinquent behaviors 144–6
developmental sequences 30
diencephalon
  engagement 71–9
  fine motor skills 68–71
  functions of 58–9
  gross motor skills 62–8
  sensory integrative processing 79–103
  sleep 59–62
Dundon, Cory 32, 68

electric toothbrushes 185
emotions 107–11
engagement 71–9
equipment
  auditory equipment 188–9
  balance bikes 179
  balloons 191–2
  baoding relaxation balls 184–5
  camping tent 183
  CapeAble weighted products 188
  chart stickers 190–1
  colored plastic film 190
  electric toothbrushes 185
  finger lights 189–90
  fitted sheets 183–4
  frozen candy 193
  Jelly Belly beans 192–3
  Lycra 172–9
  pool lights/orbs 189
  scented cotton balls 184
  sewn sweatshirt 181–3
  shaving cream 186–7
  stacking cups 185–6
  swings 166–71
  tactile spaces 180–1
  tape 192
  taste activities 192–3
  vegetable brushes 186

visual equipment 189–92
yoga balls 179–80
Erickson, C. 30

Felitti, V. J. 47
felt-safety 19–21
fine motor skills 68–71
finger lights 189–90
fitted sheets 183–4
food difficulties 35–42
foundational questions for
  assessments 147–9
frontal cortex
  delinquent behaviors 144–6
  functions of 134–5
  impulsivity 135–9
  moral reasoning 141–4
  thoughtfulness 139–41
frozen candy 193

Garner, S. 9, 23
Gobbel, Robyn 10, 15, 21–2, 78, 164
Gray, C. 79, 131, 133, 143
Greene, R. W. 20
gross motor skills 62–8

heart rate normalization 43–5
Hebb, Donald 30
hippocampus 105–6
hypothalamus 105

impulsivity 135–9
initial interactions in
  assessments 149–52
interoception 119–26

Jelly Belly beans 192–3

KALMAR app 9
  autoimmune issues activities 53–4
  breathing activities 49–50
  communication (verbal and
    non-verbal) activities 131
  delinquent behaviors activities 146
  difficulties with food activities 42
  emotions activities 111
  engagement activities
  fine motor skills activities 70–1

gross motor skills activities 67–8
heart rate normalization
    activities 44–5
impulsivity activities 139
interoception activities 125–6
moral reasoning activities 144
muscular eye movements activities
    57
relating to others activities 118–19
sense of time activities 132–3
sensory integrative processing
    activities 102–3
sleep activities 61–2
temperature regulation
    activities 46–7
thoughtfulness activities 141
waiting ability activities 132–3
weight and nutrition activities 52

Lewis, Amy 24
limbic area
    emotions 107–11
    functions of 104–6
    interoception 119–26
    regulatory state of the environment
        and social cues 111–15
    relating to others 116–19
location considerations 157–62
Lycra 172–9

MacInnes, S. 32
Maslow's hierarchy of needs 142–3
matching expectations in
    assessments 152–6
Mateos, P. 30
Maunder, Michelle 32, 68
McCane, Brenda 117
McCann, Brendan 174
Mehrabian, Albert 129
moral reasoning 141–4
muscular eye movements 54–7

nature activities 195–6
neural networks
    air traffic control analogy
        for 24–8, 29–30
    and different brain regions 24
Neurosequential Model of
    Therapeutics (NMT™) 9, 34–5

Nootboom, Nikki 38

Perry, Bruce 9, 11, 20, 22, 23,
    27, 34, 38, 78, 152, 193
pool lights/orbs 189
Porges, Stephen 19, 33
Purvis, Karyn 9, 160

Raising Kids with Big, Baffling
    Behaviors (Gobbel) 21
regulatory state of the environment
    and social cues 111–15
relating to others 116–19
resilience
    and brain regions 28–9
    therapeutic activities for 22–3
Rodríguez, A. 30

safety
    and brainstem functions 32–3
    felt-safety 19–21
    and location considerations 158
    and sense of alertness 18–20
scented cotton balls 184
sense of time 131–3
sensory integrative processing
    79–103
sewn sweatshirt 181–3
shaving cream 186–7
Simple Sparrow Sequential
    Relational Path 196–7
sleep 59–62
Smith, M. 9, 82–3, 88
Smith, R. 9
Social Stories 79, 113, 131, 1333, 143
SpIRiTed Conversations
    (podcast) 32, 68
Stackhouse, Tracy 30, 32, 78, 80, 138
stacking cups 185–6
state-dependent functioning 20–2
Sunshine, W. L. 9
swings 166–71

tactile spaces 180–1
Tanner, Jamie 107, 196
tape 192
taste activities 192–3
TBRI method 9, 116, 143, 158, 191

TCU 6
temperature regulation 45–7
thalamus 104–5
therapeutic activities
    daily activities and routines
        193–5
    nature activities 195–6
    Simple Sparrow Sequential
        Relational Path 196–7
    taste activities 192–3
therapeutic use of self 197–9
therapy animals 159–60
thoughtfulness 139–41
Trauma Lens Sensory Activity
    Response Checklist 88–100
treatment planning
    considerations 163–5

van der Kolk, Bessel 53, 120
vegetable brushes 186
visual equipment 189–92

waiting ability 131–3
Weber, J. D. 30
weight and nutrition 50–2
weighted products 188
What Happened to You? (Perry) 11
Whiting, D. 30
Winfrey, O. 20, 22, 27, 193

yoga balls 179–80